Sri K. Parvathi Kumar
Health and Harmony

Dhanishta

About the Composer

Dr. Sri K. Parvathi Kumar has been teaching various concepts of wisdom and initiating many groups into the Path of Yoga of Synthesis in India, Europe, Latin America and North America. His teachings are many and varied. They are oriented for practice and are not mere information.

Dr. Sri K. Parvathi Kumar has been honoured by the Andhra University with the title Doctor of Letters Honoris Causa, D. Lit. for all his achievements as a teacher around the world. He works actively in the economic, social and cultural fields with spirituality as the basis. He says that the spiritual practices are of value only if such practices contribute to the economic, cultural, and social welfare of humanity.

Dr. Sri K. Parvathi Kumar is a responsible householder, a professional consultant, a teacher of wisdom, healer of a certain order, and is a composer of books. He denies to himself the title of being an author, since according to him, *"Wisdom belongs to none and all belong to Wisdom"*.

The Publisher

Table of Content

Introduction 11
1. Way of Life 14
2. Educating the Sick 17
3. Life Within and Around 20
4. Factors of Disease 23
5. The Law of Evil Sharing 26
6. A Few Dimensions of Disease and Cure 29
7. The Five Ills - Their Study 31
8. Cancer and Past Ignorance 34
9. Cancer and Religion 36
10. The Blood and the Glands 38
11. Cancer 40
12. An Old Theory 43
13. Teaching and Healing 46
14. Homosexuality (1) 48
15. Homosexuality (2) 50
16. The Subtle Bodies 52
17. Worry and Irritation 55
18. The Inner Traffic 58
19. The Solar-Sacral Man 60
20. Symptoms for Diagnosis 63
21. Ethics, Morals, Medicines 65

22. Bacteria – the Effect but not the Cause 67
23. Bacteria, Life, Death 69
24. Tsunami 71
25. Simple, Healthy Living 74
26. A Simple Habit 76
27. Co-operation 78
28. Anatomy – Occult and Obvious 81
29. Holistic Healing 84
30. A Small Beginning 87
31. The Future 90
32. Endurance – a Therapy 93
33. Alchemy 96
34. Meditation 98
35. Future School of Medicine 101
36. Discipleship in Healing 104
37. Food Subtleties 107
38. Basic Health 110
39. Relevance of Astrology 113
40. Etheric Body (1) 116
41. Etheric Body (2) 119
42. Habitation and Health 122
43. Science and Theosophy 125
44. Fourfold Approach 127
45. Homeopathy 129
46. Sickness – the Doorway to Health 131
47. Vaccines 133
48. Earth – Health 135

49. The Man – His Humous Form 137
50. A Prophecy... 140
51. Post Death Healing 143
52. 3 + 5 = 8 and 9.. 146
53. Doing – Being 149
54. Karma and Health 152
55. Knowledge and Health.............................. 155
56. The Significant Shift.................................. 158
57. Threefold Pranic Supply 161
58. Upset and Set Up 164
59. The Fires in the Body................................ 167
60. Prana - Reception, Assimilation + Circulation .. 170

Introduction

"Health is wealth", is an age-old saying. Health has been the major concern at all times and much more so in the modern times where man is to cope up with the ever increasing stress and strain of living. The modern life brought along with varied developments the related ills, sicknesses, and diseases. On one side there is enormous technological development, modernized life exacting more and more from the human for the overall rapid development. On the other side there is no concurrent development in the rhythm of life giving way for many diseases, some of which are very mysterious. Man is drifting away more and more from nature in his pursuit of social and economic development. As a consequence normal natural rhythmic way of life is lost. The understanding of time, the nature and characteristics of the seasons and healthy food habits are lost. The capacity to assimilate food, which in turn maintains the vitality of the body is lost. Medicines and vitamins are being eaten as much as food. Nevertheless the growth of diseases is in geometrical progression while the inventions and innovations of medical cure are in arithmetical progression. Popular medical treatments are found to be inadequate to meet the varieties of challenges that humanity encounters in terms of diseases.

A harmonious way of living which prevents frequent falling into sickness and treatment of diseases with medicines, which are not excessively poisonous or cause more side effects than cure are the need of the hour. Men are in continuous search for alternative medicines, therapies and curative methods, due to the poisonous nature of the traditional allopathic medicine and also due to the unhealthy side affects.

Paracelsus was one of those who genuinely dedicated his life to find the cause for diseases and also to find natural medicines to cure such diseases. 500 years after his advent, Paracelsus is growing more and more relevant to the present times. His knowledge of minerals and metals, elements, and herbs seems to throw much light upon the riddle of cure. He was a genuine healer, deeply intent upon finding the right cure through right medicine and has been a source of inspiration for many. He was himself a fire philosopher, an alchemist, and a healer of a high order. In loving memory of him a group of workers in the field of health and healing decided to gather and disseminate the knowledge of health and healing as it is known in the 4 corners of the planet, which remain relatively less informed than what they deserve.

The 'Health & Healing' magazine is an activity of service that aims to help the doctors, the healers, the health workers, the sick and in general those who are interested in health and healing. The magazine proposes to give varieties of techniques of maintaining good health and also varieties of therapies for treating varied sicknesses. The cooperation of doctors, healers and health workers is the strength of the group and it is hoped that the magazine would find its effective usefulness to the humanity at large. The work is dedicated to the health of humanity. May it serve its purpose in tune with the spirit of goodwill.

1. Way of Life

A person's way of living has major impact on his health. The mental, the emotional and the physical attitudes and habits decide the degree of health or its lack of it. The attitudes of a person exist in him as seeds and sprout on a given occasion. A balanced approach to life holds the key to health. Inner harmony and poise contribute substantially to maintain stable health. In the present world covetousness, competition and the consequent jealousy are playing havoc. An average mind is affected by them. Suspicion, anger, hatred, doubt are the by-products. Fear, anxiety, depression are the further by-products. When man's mental and intellectual energies are affected by such of those mentioned heretofore good health cannot even be thought of.

Emphasis upon hygienic food, organic food etc. becomes lopsided unless man learns how to desire and how to think. He should be educated how to co-exist, co-operate and contribute to the general good, instead of his own good. Ability to adjust, adapt and live with inner poise would contribute substantially to healthy living. Frequently many fanatics of healthy food are falling sick these days. This is because healthy food alone cannot help unless they have healthy emotion and healthy mental orientation. At the same time persons with healthy mind are found to carry better health regardless of their orientation to healthy food. Furthermore in the name of health the modern man is excessively securing himself, losing the natural immunity system. In developed countries the rate and the depth of sicknesses do not seem to be far different. Their development led them to seclude themselves from their exposure to nature, weather, and atmospheric conditions. As much as one secures from the atmosphere, so much he becomes insecure vis-à-vis his resistancial powers.

Incurable diseases such as rheumatic arthritis are growing unchecked. Psychical imbalances amidst the youth are frequent. Greater dental care is counter-balanced by early loss of teeth. Medicine cannot be a solution to all this paradox. Education about the laws of nature and man's right relations with it is becoming more and more relevant. Man should be taught the human nature, the human constitution and its adjustment with the surrounding nature. Until the right way of living is learnt, the rat-race between the disease and the medicine continues to grow and health becomes ever evasive.

The modern medicine therefore should include in its education the natural laws behind health and healing.

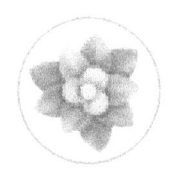

2. Educating the Sick

Health and healing has been one of the major activities of humanity. Health, sickness and healing are within the human being. The patterns of man's life, his thoughts, his emotions, his habits of eating, working and sleeping decide his health. Nature has rhythm. The functional system in man also has rhythm. When this rhythm is disturbed by man's way of living, disease manifests. Man needs to adapt to a rhythmic way of life to retain health. When he is out of rhythm, the inner functional rhythm gets disturbed. Such a disturbance is a disturbance to the flow of the stream of life.

The modern man is more and more becoming a victim of competition and the consequent jealousy, hatred and other negative emotions. He understands his sense of achievement as an act of covetousness, aggression and exploitation. This energy, in turn leads man to be manipulative. The inner consciousness gets affected by continuous manipulations and thereby invokes fear. The fear makes him to be offensive as a matter of defence. Doubt and suspicion are the by-products.

The present man is mostly bound thus by his own illusive fears, doubts, suspicions, jealousy and hatred, breeding ill health; ill health settles in the vital plane and affects the functioning of the inner life rhythm. In order to regain health, eating medicines is no solution, since through his emotional disturbance he keeps on producing disease from time to time. When one has the habit of dirtying on a daily basis, any amount of daily cleaning is no answer. He cleanses and again dirties. It is a never-ending process. In the meanwhile medicinal eating becomes part of his daily meal.

The seers of all times noticed that the disease of man is more in his behaviour. Healing is therefore to educate, to transform and thereby enable man to adopt a natural behaviour, to bring him back to normal temperament. They therefore saw the causes of diseases in the disturbed behavioural patterns. They always tried to rectify the disturbance in the patterns through suggesting the remedial measures to the way of life and remedies were also given. Thus healing was involved in teaching the normal and natural way of life. Without such remedial teachings by the healers and adoption of such teachings by the patients, the medicinal activity remains unresolved. The seers of ayurveda, homoeopathy and naturopathy strongly propounded educating the patients on these lines besides giving medical treatment.

Further, the medicines were also mostly natural

and did not have serious side effects. Whatever may be the medicinal therapy, a normal and natural way of life is necessary to be imparted by the doctors and the healers and adapted to by the patients. The source of sickness is within man. The source of healing is also within man. He needs to be educated to eliminate certain unnatural patterns to regain his health. A medical practice that imparts such education concurrently with medication is essential. All orthodox and traditional systems need to be practised with this spirit.

The above duty demands intimate interaction with the patient. Treating the patients without knowing their abnormal patterns of behaviour is a patchwork in healing, but is not healing as such.

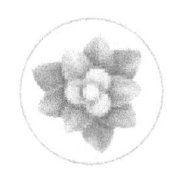

3. Life Within and Around

Man's healing energies depend upon his dynamic, positive and serviceable nature. In truth, the energies of life, health and healing are in the surroundings. Man floats in such energies. He continuously receives energies of life. Life is in him and he is in life. He is regularly a receptor of life energies for his own purpose. But he can also be a transmitter of such energies. As said earlier, a dynamic, positive and service-oriented person with love for the fellow beings can be a moderate transmitter of such healing energies. When he does so professionally, he is called a healer.

Just like a magnet transmits its energies to the surrounding iron pieces with or without its touch, a healer also can transmit energies with or without his touch. Just as magnets are used for the release of blocked energies, magnetic healing energies can also be transmitted to clear congestions, blockages and even tumors.

Sickness is generally due to a blockage of life energies. When such blockages are cleared, health is the result. From ancient times, positively oriented persons have been experimenting with these energies, which they invoked from the natural surroundings. In the East there were people who relieved people from paralysis, from blood congestion and injuries. Many soft-natured, loving but fearless individuals conducted such healing, aligning themselves with the surrounding life energies. These are generally theistic persons. Some of them had a scientific approach and some others a faith approach. Today's faith is the past science and the future science too, when explored.

Paracelsus, Mesmer, Hahnemann are some of the more known healers in the West than others, for their scientific approach. Today, man is looking for many alternative ways of natural healing in preference to eating enormous quantities of medicines. In this context, research is in progress in pockets, here and there. This needs systematization in order to be able to find ways to link up to the subtle life that surrounds us. Life enters into us not only through inhalation of oxygen, but also through the sunlight. The science of yoga says that the rays of the sun transmit life, and such life is received by man through the centre at the shoulder blades and also through the centre at the sacral. With the latest equipment, the transmission of rays into the human body and its energizing the human system can perhaps be studied seriously. Life also enters into man through food and water, besides air and light. This study of entry of life into the human system is of paramount importance, more than the study of life just within the human system. Life force should be seen as a stream flowing into and out of man. Its free flowing is his health; its congestion is his sickness.

4. Factors of Disease

Healing to ultimate perfection of health remains only an ideal. It is not practical. Many schools of health may be affirmative of such perfect healing and health. They are only high-sounding phrases, expressing their good intention. Perfect health and perfect cure are like perfect man and perfect environment. The effort towards perfection is possible while perfection is not possible. The seers of ancient times never said, "Be perfect," they only said, "Trace perfection." This is because only truth or God is perfect.

The cause for diseases is manifold and not as simple as a gullible practitioner thinks. It is not possible for man to understand the deep-seated causes, resulting in variety of diseases.

All disease is the result of lack of harmony between life and the form that envelops life. The needs of the form, the needs of the man who dwells in it and the needs of the society are at variance. This continually breeds conflict. Yoga was considered to be a discipline by which man can harmonize himself with his body and with society. But accomplishment through this means is a rare phenomenon. Very few turn out to be real yogis, while many are regretfully fake. Alignment of man with his form, his subjective feelings and objective expressions is the basic requirement of yoga, which is seldom found.

The planet wherein we all live is itself considered to be evolving and is therefore not considered as carrying ideal conditions. Astrology considers the planet Earth as a malefic planet in evolution. It is still considered awaiting its mastery. This imperfection of the planet results in imperfect bodies of the humans, besides the animals and the plants. This imperfection has an impact on health. It causes diseases.

Lack of harmony, producing what we call disease, extends to all forms of life on the planet such as animal, plant etc. The man who lives on plants and animals, is incessantly exposed to their energies. The recent mad cow disease, the bird flue and the excessive fertilizing of fields with chemicals, already produced enough disease and will continue to do so at different parts of the planet.

Man's mental and emotional activity latently and constantly produces diseases. Man's struggle for freedom and his resentment of suffering produce conflict in him, which also contributes to diseases. Man has resistance to pain, to death, to disappointment, to failures and the consequent conflict. The law of non-resistance is seldom realized as the key to health. The mentally developed man's resistance to the flow of events, his attitude of non-acceptability of life situations, is also seen as a means of disease.

Intense antagonism to disease energizes the disease, for man supplies his energy to the disease by thinking at all times of avoiding it. There is the psychological phenomenon in man to repeatedly think of what he does not want. Such continuous thinking energizes that which he does not want. This secret in man is also not known to him. Negative thinking relates to the south pole. South pole is a receptive pole; it gathers through negativism. Through negative desiring we invite that which we wish to avoid.

Thus the disease cannot be seen as the result of wrong human thoughts only. Health workers, healers and medical practitioners need to know as many dimensions as possible relating to the cause of sickness before a cure is attempted.

5. The Law of Evil Sharing

A seer of ancient times says, "Disease is the product of and is subject to three influences: first, a man's past, wherein he pays the price of ancient error; second, his inheritance, where he shares with all mankind the related tainted energy, which is of group origin and thirdly, he shares with all the natural forms that which the Lord of life imposes on his body. These three influences are called 'the ancient law of evil sharing'. This must give place some day to that 'new law of ancient dominating good', which lies behind all that God made. This law must be brought into activity by the spiritual will of man."

The ancient error mostly arises from old and static theologies, which are distorted through time and also remain fixed and rigid, regardless the changing times and related evolutions. Theologies need to be dynamic, in the sense that they should continue to be pragmatic and practicable. They should have social relevance at all times. They should find their dynamic change according to the changing living conditions. An old outfit causes confusion to an evolved structure of society. For instance, the spirit of the Vedas can be continued even in the modern life, though the structure given in ancient times may not be suitable. So is the case with Judaism, Christianity, Buddhism, Islam etc.

Man has a strong link more to the structure raised by ancient thought than to the spirit of thought. 'Love thy neighbour', 'judge not', 'pay Caesar what is his due', 'let us be fishers of men', are some of the statements coming from that great initiate Jesus the Christ, which are valid for all times, though not the structures raised by Christianity. Man's habit to hold on to the structures did not allow him to follow the spirit of the teaching. Instead of love, there is hate. Thus, theologies of all times hold humanity more by their structure than by the spirit behind. Hence they remain static. They suffer distortion and even promote erroneous points of view. This too promoted the related conflict. The error is not rectified. Today's upsurge of sex is also due to suppression in the past. Today's struggle for freedom is also due to oppression by authoritarian rule of law and of religions of the past. Man today is paying a price both for past suppression and present concept of freedom, which carries no responsibilities. Suppression of emotions causes disease; lack of regulation of emotion also causes disease. Humanity sprang from one extreme end to the other; both caused diseases. This is today's scenario.

Individually the streams of energy arising from the group are tainted and therefore, continue to affect man. The present change is an aspect of struggle to wriggle out of the past condition. Until a new balance is gained the disease continues to be rampant. It seems so. So to say, just as a woman in periods goes through many changes in her body, humanity as a whole is also going through periods of change. The will of man would eventually triumph over the disease.

6. A Few Dimensions of Disease and Cure

Healers, natural practitioners, and physicians may ponder over the following with open-mindedness:

Disease is purifying in effect. The health system within the human constitution naturally throws out the discomfort, which is seen as sickness. Symptoms of sickness are only messages of the effort of the inner auto-healing mechanism. The cure shall have to be assistant to this auto-healing system.

Cure and healing are peculiar to humanity. Humanity contacts more diseases than the plant and the animal. This is because sickness has its origin in mind, which is the speciality of man. Therefore the cure has to be more psychological than physical. This needs greater attention from the health helpers.

Disease is a process of liberation from the static state of energy. This statement needs to be thought over. Disease makes energy dynamic. A disturbance to the static state would bring in a new balance when the disturbance is met with. Many times, after cure, the patient looks more tender and radiant. The seers see disease as a means of liberation.

Disease is the state of disharmony and absence of alignment. Such disharmony exists all over. But man has to find harmony in conflict. This is gained through right understanding, right attitude and right action.

Man's approach to disease should be positive. He should gain right understanding of disease and even of death. Ignorant fight with disease is not wisdom. Fighting with disease can energize the disease.

Disease should be cured more from the psychological and emotional angles than from the symptomatic angles.

Cure has to be attempted more from the inner side of man than from the outer side. From within outwards, from more important limbs to less important limbs, from above downwards are some of the deeper cures, not the other way round. From this angle curing skin diseases requires keen attention.

7. The Five Ills - Their Study

The major group of diseases that attack mankind are essentially five, of which two predominantly affect those who are a bit advanced and a little above average, and whose intelligence is higher than that of the masses. The primary three are:
- tuberculosis
- social diseases: venereal diseases (syphilis) and
- cancer.

The other two categories that affect those who are above average are:
- heart diseases and
- nervous diseases.

These five diseases and their various subdivisions are chiefly responsible for the bulk of physical illnesses that attack humanity. There is an immediate need to gain the right grasp of the causes to give a definite assistance to medicine. This requires a study of occult anatomy, which supports the anatomy of man.

The occult scientists recognize the following as constituting the chief structure:

- the soul,
- the subtler bodies of the mind and emotions, which are simply qualified energy centers,
- the vital body with its seven major centres of force,
- the endocrine system, which is an effect of the seven centres and the determining controlling factor in the physical body of man,
- the nervous system in its three divisions,
- the blood system, and
- the glands.

The occult scientists recognize all the subsidiary organs of man as effects. The causes emanate in the functional structure, and their effects manifest in the outer structure as ills. Treatment to the effects is no treatment to the causes of illness. The determining causes in man that make him what he is are in the glands. They externalize the inner forces from the subtle side of man, which are varied and many, depending upon the current events in man's life.

The glands function or do not function as per man's evolution. Their condition depends upon man's reaction to the surrounding life. Accordingly they secrete or do not secrete. They demonstrate sufficiency, oversufficiency or deficiency.

Health or sickness is also determined, again, by the functioning of the nervous system; that is, the interlocking of the nervous system from the brain to the blood stream. This is the chief carrier of the life principle.

Glands also cause the flow of consciousness. Their functioning determines the conscious, subconscious, self-conscious, missing-conscious or super-conscious states of man.

Likewise there is a need to study the subtler bodies of man with their energy centres, and finally the soul. Any research in this direction meets the present demands of health and healing.

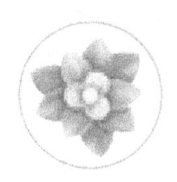

8. Cancer and Past Ignorance

Cancer is one of the most dreaded diseases and is the main preoccupation of the medical research. It would be helpful to know the psychological causes behind this disease.

Cancer is a legacy coming from the Atlantean humanity. The scourge of this disease devastated the Atlanteans. The roots of the disease are deep-seated in the emotional desire nature and are grounded in the desire body of humanity at large.

Cancer is basically a disease of inhibition and suppression of desires and emotions. The emotions of people are also strongly interlaced with sex, which was excessively suppressed through the moralistic doctrines of variety of religions. This caused suffering through suppression. While over-expression of sex leads to syphilis, suppression leads to cancer.

It is about time that man realizes that he cannot excessively suppress or excessively express any desire or emotion. Moderation and intelligent regulation of any desire is the key to health. Strong desires have their counterpart as strong aversions. One is the positive swing of emotion while the other is the negative swing of emotion. Both are extremes causing impact on the human mechanism.

Cancer has been sustained through generations and is well grounded even in the soil on which we live. Least we should understand that the germs of cancer infect the vegetable kingdom, and through the vegetable kingdom they infect the human family. It is also believed that in a similar fashion syphilis infects through the mineral kingdom.

The above said requires consideration; and also for the above stated reasons, cure is found difficult. This editorial is intended to provoke thought among those who dedicate their life to restitute health to humanity. More will be spoken on cancer in the coming editorial from the esoteric standpoint.

9. Cancer and Religion

Continuing with the basic causes of cancer disease it can be said that, apart from the emotional nature of a person and the prevalence of cancer on the planet, it signals its existence by way of over-activity or under-activity of any glandular plexus.

The over-activity or under-activity is traced by the traditional healers to the imbalance of the mind causing disturbances to the activity of a particular centre. Such imposition causes ebb and flow to the free-flowing energy system in the body. It causes too much or inadequate focus of energy at the arrested centre. One of the main causes of cancer, relating to the sacral centre, has been a well-intentioned suppression of sex life. The monastic teachings of religions and the promotion of the doctrine of celibacy in the Middle Ages led to a disturbance of the natural energy flow in the human system.

In those times people thought that sex is evil, wicked, not to be mentioned and a potential source of trouble. Normal biological reactions were violently suppressed and all thoughts of sex life were refused expression. But energy follows thought. In thought level, it is arrested. The consequence is birth and growth of tumors, and they further lead to cancer. Man should learn to transcend certain desires instead of either succumbing to them or suppressing them. Man should learn to reason out his emotions.

Similarly, religious fanaticism also leads people to cancerous states due to their foolish consecration to fanatical practices, denying the basic needs of the body. The fanatics have extreme emotional feelings and reactions, perpetuating the potential for cancer.

The same thing can be said about the violent inhibition imposed by truth seekers upon all emotional reactions and feelings. In their effort to control their desire body they resort to direct inhibition and suppression. These suppressions create a reservoir of energy drastically retained. Most of the aspirants do not have the will to transmute that retained energy into aspiration for occult growth. The consequence is cancer of stomach, of liver and sometimes of the entire area of the abdomen.

These are the fruitful areas for cancer to perpetuate.

10. The Blood and the Glands

The mystery of blood remains to be solved by the researchers of medicine. It should receive increasing attention by all who are concerned with disease, health and healing. The blood stream as also the centres or plexus, require greater attention. Their physiological effects need to be studied. When the centres are all properly developed, organized and directed, the energy which they receive from the surroundings is distributed into the physical organism. This is an important factor presently overlooked. The distribution is through the blood stream while the reception of energies is through the glandular plexus.

The blood stream is thus the agent of the glandular system. It is therefore the effect of the glandular system. The glandular working and its effect is transmitted to every part of the body by the blood stream. The blood stream thus brings certain essential elements which are known so little today, which are responsible for making man physiologically what he is, and which are also responsible for the status of the physical body and its control.

The glands receive essential elements and the blood distributes. The diseases can be either from ineffective reception of elements by the glands or from ineffective distribution by the blood stream. The blood stream also carries life. The life energy, coupled with glandular energy, penetrates the entire body and radiates into the arteries, the veins and the capillaries. If the centres do not function, the energy runs wild, becomes overactive and gets misdirected. This causes the related diseases in the related region.

An open-minded investigator may regard the possibility of the presence of the etheric centres behind the glands and may make investigations. Such an open-mindedness will give far more rapid progress. An intelligent investigator may pick up the task of studying the effects of the glands by accepting this as hypothesis. A proper study of ductless glands and of the blood stream will reveal the causes of paramount importance, which form the basis for the physical difficulties. Slowly the investigator will be led to the inevitability of the existence of the etheric centres. This will lead to inclusion of the subjective nervous system (nadis). This inclusive study will throw open the factors that are responsible for the major diseases and for obscure elements that plague humanity today. Ayurveda is one medical system that recognizes the nadis up to date.

11. Cancer

In days such as these, almost anyone is prone to cancer. Fear is the great predisposing factor for cancer, while inertia and emotionalism are the other factors. No one is as prone to cancer as the above mentioned types. A fully active life, which enables constructive engagement of mind, prevents diseases.

Excessive emotions, depressions, excessive inertia and frequent attacks of fear can be gauged before. A true healer should notice these tendencies and should suggest the necessary remedial measures in terms of work, aspirations and daily living conditions. This approach to cure needs to be thought of. This requires a personalized approach to the patients, their families and their antecedents. Once the malignant condition is established potentially, the disease of cancer cannot be cured.

Cure is only possible in the early states provided the person to be healed is fully co-operative. In occult circles it is believed that healing prayers are effective to calm down the emotions. The prayer through sound and colour therapy cleanses the aura of the persons. The healers do not direct the healing energy directly to the tissues of the cancer even if a cancerous condition is prevailing. They cleanse the emotions in the aura and transmit golden light uttering the related sound and colour. Sound and colour are seen as a therapy in the occult circles to contain and some times prevent cancer. This is a harmless practice, since the healers do not meddle with the cancerous tissues and tumors.

In the occult sense cancer is seen in the behavioural pattern, much before the transmutation of cells. Emotions do exist in humans, and such emotional forces are so heavy these days that seldom people are free from them. Since ladies are generally more emotional than males, the incidence of cancer is seen more in ladies than in males. They are not only more emotional but also have the consequent fears, anxiety and tension. Males are generally affected by such habits as smoking, drinking etc.

In the present times it cannot be ignored that there is an intensified group activity. There is certain communion of inherited group tendencies. A person who is weak in resistance attracts the impact of these group tendencies. Persons weak in mind and in vitality are prone to respond to the ills emanated from the group emotions and group thoughts. This is also one of the causes of cancer which was not so prevalent in earlier and more leisured days of life. There is increased stimulation of the body in urban places where there is massed group existence. The massed group life leads to massed cell emanation and radiation. This constant stream of energy pouring out from the body cells of massed humanity produces in certain types of people a stimulation of the structure of the body cells. This usually occurs where there is weakness in the vital body and the consequent lack of resistance. The cell defence is impaired and the result is a cancerous condition. This should be given thought. The social structure needs to be decentralized with more ventilation, breeze and vegetation for habitation.

12. An Old Theory

The physical body is visualized as a house with two communicative systems such as telephonic installations. One brings communication from outside into the house (body). The other is like a room to room telephone within the house (intercom). Mind is the telephone that brings information and through mind the information is passed into the internal communication system.

What mind brings in is the input, which is transmitted inside through the intercom within the body. The information received is analyzed by the mind according to its orientation. It can be neutral to the information. It can also be either attractive or repulsive to it. The mode of reception decides the chemistry of health. The positive reception promotes health. The negative reception promotes ill health. Discrimination to eliminate unhealthy thoughts emerging from the information gathered from the surroundings is therefore considered more as a healthy habit than a religious virtue. Entertaining them in the mind is likewise more a vice than a religious sin. Classification of this habit in terms of religion or moral is to be replaced by the science behind it. If this science is promoted man knows that it is unhealthy to indulge into extreme dislike, criticism, superiority complex etc.

The second step is to observe within the behavioural pattern the emergence of such negative emotions from within the house (body). Regardless the events outside, man feels from within the above mentioned negative emotions which should be known as deeper weeds in his own nature. Some are jealous for nothing. Some carry hatred. Some others carry critical attitude. These attitudes are true sources of sickness.

Thus the causes for ill health develop either from within or from outside as per one's reaction to a given situation. The outer causes subside faster. The inner causes do not. The two installations can thus bring in health or ill health as per the quality of thoughts produced.

The tendency to criticism, to violent dislikes and hatred, to feel superior or inferior produces acidity in majority of people. Antacids are no answer to recurring acidity. Many people today are prone to inferiority complex in relation to themselves, but to superiority complex in relation to others. All this brings in recurrently acidity.

Likewise the excessive desire to eat and drink brings in attacks of biliousness. Mostly people wake up with headache due to last night's dinner. Such people carry also yellowish face in the morning hours.

Likewise many of the common discomforts called sicknesses can be eliminated through neutralizing the existing wrong attitude in life. Such simple remedies need to be communicated than to fill the stomachs of the people with tablets of medicine.

Thus runs an old theory on medicine.

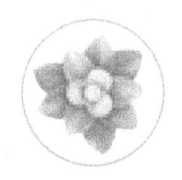

13. Teaching and Healing

Doctors and healers would do well to know that 90% of the diseases are due to wrong use of mental energy and misapplied desires. The bulk of humanity does not yet know how to use the mental and the desire energies. The human race is still very Atlantean, i.e. desire-oriented. To fulfill their desires they carry on manipulation in their thinking process. The manipulative are manipulated in due course of time. Such is the law. As long as self-propitiation exists, diseases perpetuate. Humanity at large is in conflict at the mental and emotional plane due to such continuous manipulations. The inner conflict produces incessantly diseases. However much outer cure is effected, disease repeatedly manifests as long as the inner conflict remains.

An education for a healthy living should pitch upon such new areas as 'how to think and how to desire'. The right relationship has to become once again part of human health and healing discipline. Imparting the law of right relationship therefore becomes all the more important.

There are three major laws of health, which help the present medical science to serve better the cause of health. These are indicated in the ancient scriptures. They are:

- The law of controlling and directing the will.
- The law of rhythm, which needs to be gained in terms of activity, food, rest, besides breathing and thinking. This would enable the human beings to be in harmony with nature and in equanimity with all beings. This eventually paves the way for peaceful existence.
- The law of fair distribution of material resources of the planet between the groups of humanity without controlling them for the benefit of a few. Covetousness, avarice and the related fears are dissolved when fair distribution of resources is resorted to.

The above laws should no more be seen as theosophy, religion or belief in God. The aforesaid laws should be seen as part of the science of life and health. The yoga science recognizes this fact. The patients need to be given a way of life. This is more important than diagnosing diseases and giving medicines all the time. To sum up: doctors need to be teachers also. In ancient times healers were teachers and teachers were healers too!

14. Homosexuality (1)

Homosexuality is seen in some quarters of thinkers as human development in thought. Very specious arguments are advanced to prove that this human abnormality is a sign of man becoming androgynous. These thinkers say that androgynous man or woman is gradually making appearance in evolution. Apart from these thinkers, the knowers know that this understanding is not true. The knowers know that this is one of the major problems of deep sickness, deeper than cancer, aids, and tuberculosis. Homosexuality is clearly understood as human perversion; yet they stand a great chance for a leap forward in evolution.

Homosexuality is a 'leftover' from the excesses of the human past. These beings who succumbed to the perverse habits of sex remained unsatiated. They went into unwholesome practices and became slaves of most forbidden practices. These continue to incarnate and also grow in numbers. Since they are very ancient humans on the planet they also have the related evolution through time. Their evolution permits them to make a leap forward in development if they turn at once to super-mundane and subtle aspects of life. They can turn their strong desire for sex into creativity of the highest order, which they are capable of. Spiritually they are understood to be senior inhabitants of the planet and they can claim back their status as creators to help humanity. Through time these ancient souls have gained enormous will, besides experience of life through exposure. Their will has the ability to manifest, which through perversion took to wrong direction. They need to be appropriately and subtly addressed of their innate abilities. Carefully and caressingly they should be directed to constructive thinking. This results in resurrection of their will.

Solution is to be given to them intelligently by doctors and psychiatrists, revealing their strength to them. These are the cases where a great strength remains inversed as a great weakness. This needs to be reversed. It is a noble act that requires attention by the medical profession.

15. Homosexuality (2)

Continuing with the theme of homosexuality, which is a 'leftover' from the excesses of Lemurian times, an inherited taint, it may be said that there is today 'imitative homosexuality' prevailing in the human community. In fact, the imitative homosexuality is far more in numbers than the original. The originals stand a good chance by reorientation to goodwill, but the duplicates do not have that chance. They have only an option to drop from such evil habits. The solution to them is to get away from such imitations. They indulge through their imitation into wild imagination and prurient curiosity. These tainted people are baser in their nature and have powerful physical bodies and ugly sex orientations. Their psychology leads them to give birth to sodomites and lesbians. These sicknesses are deep and generally cannot be retrieved. They are in a difficult situation. So the psychologists are dealing with them. They are subjects of deep pity and commiseration and need humanitarian consideration.

Much light needs to be thrown upon this problem, since a large number of people are called upon to face it. The goodwill workers, physicians, social workers, psychologists and all allied workers meet with this problem. They would do well to know the originals and the imitative ones.

The inherent taints spoken of in the editorials before, such as excessive desires for material, for sex, need to be seen as the root cause for all the major sicknesses on the planet. Humanity carries these taints over many generations, and the physicians need to recognize it. It would be an interesting experiment if these various inherent difficulties of mankind are understood and their consequent diseases are recognized. It is these original impulses, which need to be treated, but not the peripheral manifestations. That is the real challenge for the medical service today.

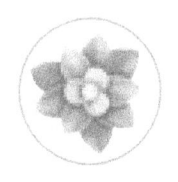

16. The Subtle Bodies

It is time that the medical science as a whole awakens and moves towards study of the vital body, emotional body and etheric body, which relate to human vitality, circulation of life force and digestive system. Enough is known to the medical science regarding the concrete facts of the dense physical body. The functions of vitality conducted by the organs of respiration and of circulation by the heart, the circulatory and the nervous system are closely related. They need to be further studied.

The faculties of respiration and of sleep are closely related. If respiration is affected, sleep is affected and the brain is affected. Brain is the mind's organ, thus mind is affected. Consequently man is confused. Thus the effect of respiration has its chain action and it needs to be recognized.

Similarly, the heart and its circulatory system and the nervous system are of paramount importance. The proper functioning of the heart, the circulatory system and the nervous system assimilates the vitality produced by the respiratory activity. The vitality is transmitted through the blood stream and the nervous network. In turn, it affects the organs of assimilation and elimination conducted by the stomach and bowels. When the stomach and bowels are affected, various diseases emerge below the diaphragm.

How many physicians today inquire about sleep when a patient narrates some discomfort? How many check up the pulse to note the circulatory aspect of life force? How many interrelate the stomach with heart and brain? That the brain and the respiratory activity are interrelated is very well known in yoga, ayurveda and in many ancient health sciences. In turn they are related to the circulatory and nervous systems. Whatever and wherever the discomfort may be, the entire triplicity of the human system needs to be checked to find the cause of disease. This is possible only when a holistic approach is made to study the functional aspect of the physical body represented by the etheric, emotional and vital bodies. This necessitates study of the etheric body, vital body and emotional body of human beings.

The entire human activity is polarized towards desire, causing vigorous movement of emotions and the related disturbance to the emotional body and affecting the nervous system. When the emotional body is thus disturbed, the etheric body does not function properly, in the sense it does not transmit sufficiently prana to the physical body. When prana, the life force, is not well supplied, the organs of assimilation and elimination do not function well. When elimination and assimilation do not function well, it produces carbon and affects respiratory organs, which would lead to mental strain and eventual collapse, leading to depressions, absentmindedness and sleeplessness.

The physician therefore has to gently enquire into the thought and desire patterns of a patient besides noting the symptoms. Such was the ancient way of healing. Such should be again the New Age healing.

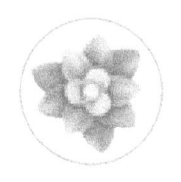

17. Worry and Irritation

Worry and irritation should be seen as one of the major causes for sickness by the medical profession.

Today life has become more uncertain than before and the uncertainty stimulates worry. It causes irritation. Everyone is involved in the world's uncertainty. The difference is in degree. It disturbs the life current.

There is excessive intercommunication between people, consequently there is little solitude. Even in the rare moments of solitude man's mind is preoccupied about others or about the problems surrounding him. Either physically or mentally man is massed. Consequently mass energy prevails over the individual energy. The quality of the energy qualitatively affects the person. Quantitative effect is also there.

Many carry with them others' sufferings and unconsciously develop seeds through pity. Pity is negative energy while sympathy is positive. Negative energy is receptive. Therefore the contagion happens. There is truth in this.

Weak-minded people 'tune in' to others' emotional conditions and mental attitudes, causing constant disturbance to their own energy leading to sickness. To their own engrossing worries they add others' worries also.

People are also affected by the television, radio, newspapers and recently internet, which transmit a lot of negative news of war, violence, deaths, accidents, natural calamities, crises etc.

Today, to face up to life is not easy unless one insulates himself against such onslaught of negative energy. This negative energy can be comprehended by any average thinker of the day. According to a Master of Wisdom this is an 'imperil' - they are perilous and serious.

The ancient healers knew that worry and irritation lower the vitality of a person to such a point where he is vulnerable to diseases.

Secondly, worry and irritation are infectious from the astral point; in the sense, it will affect the breathing. People with worry and irritation cannot breathe freely, bringing in circulatory diseases. Incomplete breathing also affects the flow of energy through nerves.

A deeply worried person at home spreads epidemic. Today, such people are many spreading the epidemic planetarily. Worry and irritation have inflammatory effect. They cause the inflammation of variety of limbs.

Lastly the person affected by worry and irritation is blurred of his vision in terms of sight and comprehension.

These are a few to mention. The physician would do well to give psychological antidote to this energy of worry and irritation.

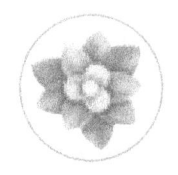

18. The Inner Traffic

"Where there is more traffic, there are more accidents. Traffic coupled with speed causes greater accidents," says a seer in relation to health. From the seers' standpoint the body is full of lines of force and these lines of force cross each other forming the traffic centres. Unless the traffic signals are followed, accidents happen. These traffic signals are the age-old health regulations.

From the seers' standpoint the physical body is an automaton run by the etheric body, which is composed entirely of lines of force; and where these lines of force cross each other, they form centres of energy. Where more lines of force cross each other, they form major centres. Thus in the etheric body there are 7 major centres, 21 minor centres and 49 smaller centres. These centres of energy and lines of force run the automaton, the physical body.

When there is free flow of force through the etheric body to the dense physical body, the scope for signals and disease is little. Whenever there is disturbance to the equilibrium, there is over or under stimulation of energy, and such disequilibrium leads into the dense physical body. The disequilibrium can be from the environing world or from the personality of man. The congestion in the human vehicle is due to inappropriate flow of forces and energy via the etheric body to the physical body.

The first impact of such congestion is generally at the lungs or at the throat and head. Not infrequently the congestion settles in the stomach. It is for this reason the human attitude towards life is as important as the environing condition. The attitude recommended is one of dynamic passivity, while the humans are generally aggressive, competitive and jealous. A balanced, poised, stable mind is a precious shield for health as well. The emotional and aggressive ones are generally left unshielded to the prevailing conditions.

19. The Solar-Sacral Man

The new medical science will be substantially built upon the science of the etheric centres in man. Upon this knowledge all diagnosis and cure will be based. The endocrinologist of the medical science is today glimpsing into the possibilities of such centres as he attempts to balance the glandular system and as he studies the relation of the glands to the blood stream. Endocrinology is today engaged with the relation of the blood stream to the glands, and is also deeply engaged in balancing the glandular system. The study is today focused upon the character of many glands and the attitudinal predisposition of many patients. The discovery is running towards considering the basis for the functioning of the glandular plexus. The real value in such study is deemed worthy. Much however remains to be discovered before it will be really safe to work with the glands.

Today much distress to the physical body is due to congestion in the etheric body arising from the astral (desire) plane. The unfulfilled desires cause congestion in the etheric body. The non-fulfillment of desires creates pressure in the subtle (etheric) body. And there is no point of outlet to such desires. Every desire emanates a particular type of etheric force and unless it passes through, the congestion happens. The free play between the etheric body and the physical body results in free flow and passage of the forces involving the nerve ganglia and the endocrine system.

The 7 major glands in the human body should enable the free flow of human thought and desire, without which glandular imbalance is given birth to. This should never be forgotten. The functioning of the glands has its roots in the condition of the etheric centres. The functioning of these centres in turn depends upon the free flow of thoughts and desires. This is where man is advised to entertain desirable thoughts and desires only. When his thoughts and desires remain unfulfilled for one reason or the other, he is opening doors for etheric congestion and the related glandular imbalances as also the consequent endocrinal disturbances.

All the above will definitely be considered and discovered in the coming age. The new medical science will be outstandingly built upon this knowledge.

The bulk of humanity today is desire-oriented. They need to learn much in matters of 'how to think and what to desire'. Men of wisdom call this present humanity 'solar-sacral people'. They need to ascend towards clean thinking. The measures for the needed ascent are available in the wisdom science. Thus, the medical science once again approaches the wisdom science for better solutions. This seems to be the future.

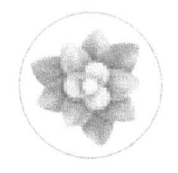

20. Symptoms for Diagnosis

In the contemporary world manipulation has become common. Manipulations produce their consequent ill health and undesirable effects. All manipulation is selfish and is for personal ends. It disturbs the sacral centre and consequently gastric and intestinal disorders emerge. The various stomach troubles, which devastate the civilized humanity far more than the savage races, are due to the clever manipulations of the human brain. In fact, such manipulations also cause brain disorders of low order.

Manipulative actions cause agitation. Regular attack of agitation disturbs the vital body producing discomforts and the disease in the stomach. Once the stomach is thus regularly affected, it affects the pancreas, the gall bladder and it also results in indigestion. Today few people in the human race are free from indigestion, undesirable gastric conditions and troubles connected with the gall bladder. Attacks of biliousness are also frequent.

Humanity is conditioned by desire: good, selfish, wrong, and even by spiritual desire. Desire of any kind galvanizes the energies around the solar plexus. Any desire makes one ambitious. Consequently, the solar plexus connected to the stomach is the most disturbed centre in the body. It has thus become the basic cause of the majority of stomach complaints and troubles connected with the liver.

The entire area immediately below the diaphragm is in a constant state of turmoil for an average man due to the unfulfilled ambitions, which have their basis in desire. To fulfil them he succumbs to manipulations. Unless humanity knows the cost of manipulations it will continue to suffer the disorders of stomach, intestine, liver and pancreas. It is time for the medical profession to recognize this symptom in its effort to diagnose the disease.

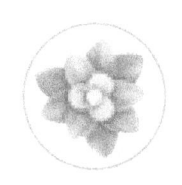

21. Ethics, Morals, Medicines

Sleeplessness and respiratory difficulties are known to arise from violent emotional attitudes. Intense worry, prolonged irritation, the tendency to criticize, to violent dislikes and to hatreds contribute to hyperacidity, gastric problems and respiratory difficulties leading to sleeplessness. When such condition continues it could lead to diseases of the brain of the lower order.

When emotions are improperly directed, diseases emerge below the diaphragm. When the will is not properly used, diseases emerge above the diaphragm. Medical science therefore should eventually seek solution through simpler methods to rectify the behavioural aspects of the patient than to get into the complexity of drugs and operations. The energy system and its quality can be better changed through adaption to better patterns of life. Understanding of right use of energies offers a better scope of cure than antibiotics, cortisone and other powerful poisonous medicines.

By the development of goodwill comes the healing of the diseases of the respiratory tract, lungs and throat. Goodwill is good intention and good motive in all that one does. It generates energies to heal and even to stabilize the brain cells. It cures obsessions and insanities. The ancients, especially the yogis, knew that goodwill can even ensure longevity of life. Yogis of the past could even extend their life through goodwill until they finished their work. As per yoga, goodwill activates life and nourishes the brain cells and the respiratory system.

Likewise the ancients also strongly advised appropriate use of intelligence to enable appropriate functioning of the organs below the diaphragm.

Consciously the ancients promoted a way of life for human society where goodwill and appropriate use of intelligence were the benchmarks. Unconsciously religious faith promotes the same by way of morals and ethics. The science behind the morals and the ethics holds the clue for many diseases of humanity. The medical science needs to explore them through scientific approach.

22. Bacteria – the Effect but not the Cause

The theories held as to the origin of diseases and recognition of bacteria and germs are largely correct. But the bacteria are the result and not the cause. The cause is hidden in the history of the planet and of mankind. Man and the planet, it should be remembered, are millions of years of age. Civilization goes back to Atlantean and Lemurian ages, which the occult science puts at over 15 million years and above. Man himself is traced to 18 million years and the planet 30 million years. There were times when man lived intimately with animal, plant and the rock. He related himself closely to the 3 lower kingdoms. He thus lived, loved, and experienced. The human bodies absorbed many things from many surroundings, which continue to form part of the cells of the physical body. This brings with them predisposition and the inherent tendencies which the past history endowed on them.

Thus the physical bodies in which human beings live are constructed with very old matter, and the substance of the body is tainted by the history of man and of the planet. This remains a mystery to man and to science.

People entertain a fallacy that the ancient races were all free from disease and from contamination and unhealthy living conditions. They were carrying their own contamination, unhealthy living conditions, unhealthy habits and the consequent diseases. In the infancy of the race, there was the great ignorance of mismating, promiscuity and a host of perversions giving birth to variety of bacteria, germs and other organisms. Thus the latter are the effects of the past human activity. It should therefore be understood that there cannot be a completely healthy physical body on the planet.

To quote from an old scripture, "Earth took its toll of human pollution and impurity. Earth to earth, i.e. living forms merge in the earth and draw from the earth. Thus evil life entered the pristine cleanliness of the ancient mother. Deep in the soil the evil lies, emerging into form from time to time. Only fire and suffering can cleanse the mother of the evil which her children have given unto her." The bacteria are the effect of it and are today seen as the cause.

23. Bacteria, Life, Death

Science teaches that the living as well as dead organisms of both, man and animal, are swarming with bacteria of a hundred varieties. The science says that we are threatened with an invasion of microbes. With every breath we draw from outside and from within also, we are threatened by leucomaines, aerobes, anaerobes etc.

But the occult science says that our body as well as those of animals, plants and even stones, are themselves all together built up of such bacteria! Science is now on its way to discoveries that will go far towards corroborating the theory of occultists. Chemistry and physiology would open the doors to mankind to great physical truths. The identity between animal bodies and human bodies, between plant bodies and man's body would be comprehended. The physical and chemical constituents of all beings would be found identical. The matter that composes the ox and the form of man would be found to be of no difference in their chemical composition. Not only the chemical compounds, but also the infinitesimal invisible lives that compose the atoms of the bodies of every form are the same as per the occult science.

Every particle, whether organic or inorganic, is a life, says the occult science. It also says that every atom and every molecule in the universe is life-giving and death-giving too to the form, inasmuch as it builds by aggregation the ephemeral vehicles.

It creates and kills. It is self-generating and self-destroying every second in time and space. Such is the understanding of bacteria in the occult science, which regards them as fiery lives that manifest the mysteries of life. They are countless myriads of lives. They are invisible too. They are the means for the manifestation of what is termed as the life force in the body.

The fiery lives that build the human body and maintain it, they also eventually destroy the body.

The bacteria, therefore, need to be studied further than what is presently understood. The fire and the life in the bacteria need to be comprehended.

24. Tsunami

Man is the president; mind is the secretary. Man's thought patterns and behaviour are his lady. The senses are the assistants to the secretary. The body is the servant. It is not the man that decides the activity; it is the lady. She works more through the secretary and not the president (the man). He remains a witness, while his lady uses his organization. It is the lady's rule that prevails! Behaviour prevails over knowledge.

Thus, mind is more a transmitter of thoughts and desires (the lady) generated from the man. Mind (the secretary) is not the one that decides. The man is also not the one that decides. It is mostly the lady (the settled pattern of thoughts and desires) that decides. Thoughts occur but people think that they think. It is not true. Thoughts occur even if people don't want to think. In fact, what man does not want to think, he thinks more! Thoughts flow through the mind and not from the mind. The transmission needs to be of even flow. Then the mind remains healthy. But the lady is covetous, jealous, aggressive and speedy. Then there is flood of thoughts. The lady also suffers from fear, doubt and suspicion. Then the flow is feeble. Thus uneven flow of energies happens as per the inconsistencies of the lady (behaviour). Then the system gets unhealthy.

If healthy thoughts flow, mind becomes healthier and it passes health to the senses and the body. If thoughts are not healthy, it passes unhealthy energy to the senses and the body: 'Energy follows thought'. Right thoughts bring in right energy, other thoughts bring in other energies.

Besides, rhythmic flow of thoughts brings in greater life force because life moves in rhythm. If there is rush of flow at one time and meek flow at another time, mind and its organization get affected. If there is frequent disturbance of voltage, the electrical equipment gets damaged; likewise, the body gets damaged. Rhythm is important for the life force. Heartbeat, blood circulation, breathing and respiration are all rhythmic, if we observe. This rhythm is disturbed by the uneven flow of thoughts. It is also disturbed by thoughts of hate, malice, jealousy, anger and any strong emotion.

This importance of rhythmic and healthy flow of thoughts is little realized by the modern people who are in excessive activity with no rhythm vis-à-vis sleep, work, food and rest. Modern life is so stressful that rhythm is frequently disturbed. Frequent disturbance to rhythm would result in much ill health, including mental ill health.

Man's quest for material amassment is leading him to overlook all important life rhythms. The result is gradual imbalance in the rhythmic flow of energy through mind. The law of rhythm is a mental law. There is widespread infringement of this law today. The scriptures compare the flow of thoughts to the flow of waves to the shore. There is a rhythm in their flow; there is a song in their movement. When the song of waves is disturbed, it is like a tsunami. Today there are a lot of mental tsunamis, which we need to cognize and rectify. We are worried about the physical tsunami. Mental tsunami is subtle, unnoticeable and more dangerous than oceanic tsunami.

Mental sickness is thus due to excessive arrhythmic flow of thoughts through mind. It can also be due to lack of flow of thoughts, which is the twin brother of the excessive flow. The overflow and the lack of flow are the obverse and reverse of the coin.

The medical profession needs to assert for social laws to restore equanimity between work, social activity and sleep. This basic triangle cannot be disturbed through mania for more work, more money and more power. This is the need of the hour. "Prevention is better than cure", says the noble profession of medicine.

25. Simple, Healthy Living

From ancient times in Himalayas there has been a simple way of healthy living. A short pranayama (breathing exercise) in the morning, not longer than 5 minutes, intake of vegetables, fruits, milk and cereals, an appropriate footwear while moving, a positive attitude of mind to receive the events of the day form part of the daily routine. Meat, wines and opium are seen as enemies to health. Many till date follow this dietary system in the remote valleys of the Himalayas. These simple mountain dwellers have much better health than the citizens of global cities and towns.

Among the vegetables, asparagus, celery and garlic are particularly avoided. They are considered as medicines and are used when there is disturbance to health. Exposure to sunlight, bathing in river streams, drinking spring water, sitting around fireplaces, are also part of daily life to have better psychic energy.

It is common knowledge among the people in these valleys, and they distinguish nature with its vegetation as life giver, preserver, restorer and even as destroyer.

They tend to use nature's products in all these four directions, as per the hour of need.

One can easily strengthen the action of a vegetable substance by increasing the metalization of the soil. These dwellers of the mountains know the related technique and cultivate.

Much knowledge of health and healing exists even today in such valleys, which is useful for scientific study and for simple curative techniques. Sometimes we need to be simpler to find solutions to complicated cures. Many times better health goes in association with simple and natural living. May the scientific age lead humanity towards simplicity.

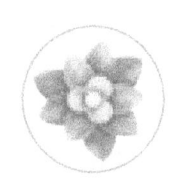

26. A Simple Habit

It is refreshing to think afresh of food. Certainly the wisest course is to partake in food, when the body has need of it. It is equally wise to take food only twice daily. It is considered sufficient if man eats twice, spread over the day. People think that it is difficult to follow this rule. It is certainly not difficult if one is intent upon it. Eating many times during the day may be a fashion but is certainly not healthy. The stomach should be given work at definite hours, but not at any time as one pleases. It is most harmful to consume food without definite hours and without need. Eating for social purpose is not acceptable to the stomach. The wise do not disturb the rhythm of the stomach. It is as consequential as the disturbance to rhythm of the heart.

Rhythmic and orderly life is not something shameful and avoidable. Let not the excessive socialization and modernization result in disturbing the rhythm of the body. One must know and carefully protect the apparatus called the human body, which is built through ages.

It is incorrect to believe that man needs a lot of food. All that he needs is little but qualitative food. One should avoid acids and artificial preparations. The modern aerated cool drinks that substitute the natural fruit juice and drinks are all harmful. Decaying butter and stored cheese are even more harmful.

Blessed is the one who burdens not himself with food. The modern man is least educated in these lines. When fundamentals of health are at stake diseases are bound to emerge. The fast food centres, running breakfasts, junk food of fashion as well as artificial drinks have taken the humanity away from health. Natural normal food, which is qualitative, is rare to find. Rhythm is almost absent.

It is time that the medical profession educates the society at large as to the need for rhythmic eating and the need for simple qualitative food in modest quantities.

27. Co-operation

The well-being of humanity is envisioned as a possibility when the work of the doctor and the surgeon would be supplemented by the analysis and conclusions of the psychologist and when the power of right thought comes in as an aid. Then and only then we will enter into a new era of well-being of human beings. To the various categories of sicknesses various healing agencies should be added for accomplishing the tasks. The treatment has to be for the whole man and should not be limited to the parts in which the doctors are specialized. There should also be the ability to comprehend the nature of energy of the patient, a correct appreciation of his endocrine system, its glands and their subtle relationship.

Presently there is no coherence between
- physicians and surgeons, orthodox and academic,
- neurologists, psychologists and psychiatrists,
- homoeopaths, naturopaths, ayurvedic doctors, and such alternative medical practitioners,
- healers and health workers.

There is much antagonistic thinking and mutual criticism between these groups instead of loving understanding and integration of strengths. Every system has its strengths and weaknesses and no single system is a complete answer to the present state of diseases. All are interdependent but not independent. This needs to be realized. To realize this, the groups should have a large heart but not a narrow mind.

It is the inability of these groups to recognize the good in the other groups striving for the well-being of humanity, which makes it almost impossible to usher in the holistic treatment. Every pioneering idea has to batter itself against the existing crystallized thought forms. The dead weight of preconceived and prejudiced views pulls back the pioneerism of a well-intentioned few. The field of medicine is so difficult that fear enters and destroys every new and progressive idea. The gulf between the old and established and the new, needs much bridging through time.

Orthodox medicine is slow to accept other systems. At times it is too slow to accept the strengths of other systems. It is slow because the risk to the humans is too great to accept anything which is not scientific and statistically proven. It cannot afford to make experiments. But the facts are that there is already substantial experimentation happening, even within the orthodox medical practice. Why not be open for other experimentation also?

Orthodox medicine, with all its failures, has however advanced by leaps and bounds. The science of electricity and light therapy, the incessant research, the space medicine are all to its credit. They are ever trying newer approaches to diseases.

The approach of the mental healers and alternative medicine has not proceeded so helpfully. This is largely their fault. They hurt their own cause owing to the large claims, which they make, and to their antagonism towards orthodox medicine. Many of their cures are faith cures. Their claims of cures are both correct and incorrect. They need to keep a record of not only their successes but also of their failures. But they too have strengths where orthodox medicine is weak.

The middle way of compromise and of mutual co-operation is ever the wisest. This is a lesson much needed today in every department of human thinking.

28. Anatomy – Occult and Obvious

Comprehension of two aspects of the human body will greatly facilitate an increasing sensitivity and clearer perception of the body's health condition.

The two aspects are:

- mass of knowledge and information about the physical body, which is accumulated down the ages by men of science and which is largely proven,
- a constantly growing understanding of the nature of the etheric body, of the etheric centres, and of the transmission and circulation of energies of awareness besides the energies of life.

The medical profession may have to realize one subtle factor. The World War II tremendously increased the nervous sensitivity and also the capacity for nervous reactions. This increased nervous receptivity is growing to abnormal levels, and the results are sad. The nervous apparatus of the average Westerner is unstable and is leading to much nervous disorder. A greater measure of mistrust, doubt, suspicion, hatred, jealousy and fear is found in the materially advanced societies of the West than in the other societies which are relatively poor.

The orthodox physician is more or less well informed of the physical anatomy of man while the metaphysical healer carries knowledge of the occult anatomy of man where the functioning of the force of intelligence and its quality is given greater emphasis. Man is the result of two streams of energy flowing through him: one is the stream of life, the other is the stream of light (awareness, rational thinking, acting, perceiving etc). Health is a product of right thought, right action, right food and sleep. The science of medicine finds its solutions when man as a whole is considered. That is, his attitude towards work and society, the thoughts he entertains, the food he takes in, his rhythm of sleep, action, exercise and food etc.

The physician and the metaphysician should necessarily come together. Both have much to do together because the work of one penetrates into the other. The two are interdependent. The subtle and the intangible should meet the obvious and the tangible. This is the future. The metaphysician is helpless without the physician and vice versa.

More often the physician complains that the metaphysicians are charlatans. But charlatans also exist among physicians. They are few in number in both groups. They are to be avoided in any case. The sincere investigators that have immense love for humanity can be found in both groups. They should come together dispelling mutual fears to find sensible and complete solutions to meet the needs of human health.

29. Holistic Healing

Time has come that doctors and healers come together to heal. Healers can work supplementary to the orthodox cure of doctors. The results relating to the work on both sides can be carefully watched and noted. A group can be formed experimentally with defined areas of operation. The group may consist of:

a) an orthodox doctor who is reputed and open to alternative therapies.

b) a pranic healer who can consciously transmit pranic energies from his palms without touching the patients. He should be able to feel the areas of congestion of prana in the body and the related etheric centres.

c) an astrologer who is well versed in medical astrology and also in psychology of the patient as indicated by his astrological chart. He should also be well versed in the karma aspect of the patient through astrology. He should also fairly know the periodicity, the bio-resonance of the patient.

d) a yoga practitioner who can give simple remedial breathing and asana techniques, besides suggesting the water baths, mud baths etc.

e) a colour and sound healer who should be able to suggest the right colour and sound therapy to assist the vital body and the inflow of prana into the patient's system.

Such group should be lead by the orthodox doctor, who basically diagnoses and determines the sickness. Under his leadership others need to work. The treatment has to be given on a consultative basis.

Such a group can be more effective in relation to the present requirements of medical treatment. In ancient times a doctor carried all this knowledge in him. Hippocrates, the father of the orthodox medicine, suggested astrological knowledge to the doctors. He emphasized upon the time dimension for cure. Paracelsus emphasized upon the time, the seasons and even the places for cure. Pioneering research institutions in medicine need to think of this new approach to healing.

The formation of such a group for healing should be understood as an experiment in goodwill. The work should be carried on with certain simple rules. The learning process should be given due time. How to work together can be known fairly in two and a half years. The group should be open for changes to function for the better. Record should be kept of the experiments for guidance. Patient's cooperation is also necessary, and for this reason the patient should also be informed of this experiment of holistic healing.

Patients who are not expected to live and those who have terminal diseases should not be considered for this work initially, so that the morale of the group is not affected. Likewise, a patient should not be dropped if he gets worse; instead, a different technique can be chosen.

This is a research project, worth to be attempted in order to meet the New Age challenges – a project for holistic healing.

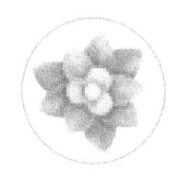

30. A Small Beginning

Humanity cannot do without its doctors, surgeons and hospitals. It will be so for the centuries to come. Modern medicine is into a great activity of research and innovation, but barriers are erected by excessive specialization, preventing new schools of thought. The new schools consist of dieticians, naturopaths, homoeopaths, ayurvedic doctors plus many others. No one is completely clear about the whole story of human health and disease. The alternative medicine claims 'a universal cure-all' and their advocates claim definiteness, sureness and certainty, which only shows many times their ignorance and arrogance. By their loudly shouted sureties they have definitely damaged their cause and consequently the modern medicine raised its barriers even higher to be separative. The alternative system, though vaguely, considers the etheric body and the etheric centres. The orthodox medicine is not open even to consider the possibilities of such etheric existence.

It is essential that in the days to come medical men should realize that disease in the physical body is incidental to the wrong internal condition. Until the true nature of the inner man, his constitution, its powers and its field of influence is comprehended, scientific cures are not possible. The medical science needs to be built around certain major premises in the near future. They are:

1. Preventive medicine will be the goal, producing the attempt to keep the body in proper balanced order.

2. Sound sanitation and the providing of healthy conditions will be regarded as essential.

3. The supply of the right chemical properties to the physical body will be studied as a science of chemistry, which is yet in its infancy, though it is becoming a flourishing infant.

4. An understanding of the laws of vitality will be regarded of prime importance, and of this, the emphasis placed today on vitamins and on the influence of the sun are wholesome indications.

5. The use of the mind will be regarded above everything else as a factor of major importance. The mind will be seen as the prime influence in regard to the centres, for people will be taught to work on their centres through mental power, and thus produce a right reaction from the endocrine system. This will necessarily involve the right direction of thought to a centre or the withdrawal of attention from a centre with the

consequent effect upon the glandular system. This will all be based upon the occult law that 'energy follows thought'.

6. The perfect healing combination is that of the medical man and the spiritual healer, each working in his own field and both having faith in each other; but this is not now the case. There is no need to call in divine aid to set bones, which the surgeon is well equipped to do or to clear up infection, which the physician knows well how to handle.

The healer can help and can hasten the process, but the orthodox physician can also hasten the work of the healer. Both groups need each other.

This is the view of the wise in the present context, which needs to be given a thought and a small beginning.

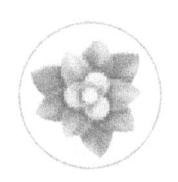

31. The Future

The treatments for sickness cannot be the same for all. The diseases of the masses, of average citizens, of the intelligentsia and of religious people differ widely, not so much in their physical expression, but in their psychological condition. For example, a bloated stomach can be due to non-digestion of food or due to fears and uncertainties, and can also be due to anxieties and irritations. A bloated stomach could also be the result of unfulfilled emotions and aspirations. There are varieties of psychological reasons for stomach imbalance.

This is a point to be cognized by an average healer. He needs to grasp these distinctions and gauge the point in evolution of each patient, which he or she may have reached. Some need to be dealt with at the psychological plane, while others may have to be dealt with at the emotional plane. Some may need just a physical cure.

If the same discomforts are repeatedly reported the healer should think deeper than routine treatment. Deeper diagnosis does not mean always more tests,

X-rays, electrocardiograms etc. It means to give more time to the patient, more interactions, seeking more information at a deeper level than just at superficial social levels.

Palliatives and ameliorating applications may eliminate present undesirable conditions; but they build up again and again in psychologically and emotionally disturbed persons. These psychological imbalances shall have to be studied in terms of attitude of mind, inhibitions, complexes, unknown fears, morbid conditions and neurotic disturbances. In all such cases, more time, more attention and a friendlier attitude are desirable from the healer.

The healing practitioner should be able to absorb and dispel through interaction and conversation the negative energy in such persons and also fill them with positive dynamic energy. Through talk the healing practitioner should be able to revitalize the devitalized patients. This requires humour and cheerfulness as a quality in the healing practitioner. The patient should leave the doctor's chamber with a better mind, a solaced and comforted mind. This is needed from the healing practitioners and doctors, who are mostly officious and air either seriousness or unfriendliness.

Psychologically positive energies should naturally emerge from a healer. This would result in a friendly atmosphere where the patient feels comforted. It is a paradox today that many psychologists turn out to be patients after a decade, by means of their work. This is because they absorb the patient's negative energy but do not know how to neutralize it within them. The key is humour, cheer, friendliness, relaxation exercises and even meditations with colour, sound, symbol etc.

Much of the psychological healing can be done by the patient himself if right colour, symbol or sound is given to him with a technique to contemplate. This is the future.

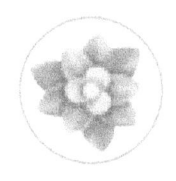

32. Endurance – a Therapy

Much medicinal work can be dispensed with if man is taught how he should plan his food, work and rest. This is a fundamental aspect of living that is missing in the so-called developed world.

Most of the sicknesses emerge in the stomach. The stomach is disturbed due to varieties of agitation. And man today is full of agitation, over-activity and the related stress of temper. The fear of the future and the sense of insecurity are reaching greater heights, and man is galvanized into hyperactivity that affects the gall duct, the gall bladder, the pancreas and the stomach. No one seems to be today an exception to these problems. The growing indigestion and the consequent gastric condition are far too common. 9 out of 10 persons seem to be constipated. Constipation has become a common sickness of the civilized society. Just as man grips everything within his reach, the solar plexus seems to grip all that is produced in the stomach.

Stomachic physical plane disorders are closely tied up with the disproportionate desire for eating, drinking of all that is desired. Little caution is exercised by the average man of the consequence of such indiscrete eating and drinking. Attacks of biliousness have become so common due to such fundamental ignorance.

The prevalent wrong attitudes to life and to people need to be noticed as causes for the stomach ills of the civilized people. Many in the civilized world do not even care to know the ultimate impact of that which they eat, drink, speak and think.

Pollution in the aspects of eating, drinking, speaking and thinking leads to restless nights. Man needs to understand that when he cannot really sleep well, it means he has a lot to rectify in him in these normal, simple, daily activities.

Eating medicines for every discomfort is yet another dimension to ignorance. Aspirin for headache, Crosin for fever, purgatives for defecation, enzymes for digestion and discharge of gas, tablets for sleeping seem to be the fashion. Many middle-aged men and women take painkillers to relieve themselves temporarily from pains. This is a dangerous habit that kills the natural resistance to disease and makes the system totally dependent on medicines.

Much of the body discomfort can be cured by sheer endurance. Endurance is also a curative technique for many acute discomforts. Man carries a healing system within himself. He should allow the system to restore normalcy. He should be educated to let the system function and support such system with appropriate intake of water and food.

Educating the common man in natural health and healing is a major work that needs to be done by the health workers. This would help avoiding, wherever possible, eating of medicines. It is time that man thinks of normal and natural methods for restoring health.

'Sickness that is not curable may be endured.'

33. Alchemy

The heat of the physical plane existence in the mounting crises of the world makes it almost impossible to think of even good health, forgetting for the moment perfect health. Perfect health is almost next to impossibility. The present physical bodies cannot cope up with the stress and strain presented by the ambitious human activity. Such is the astral desire and the related miasma that the forces in the body are struggling to have health. Astral desire, corruption and the foul cesspools of the lower levels of mental desires infect all. Lucky if one escapes from the onslaught of the sticky astral energy prevailing over humanity!

With weak and sensitive human bodies much fight and struggle are conducted. Failure, pain, tension, labour, followed by racked nerves, tired head, ached heart, are too common to be ignored. Living has become a struggle for rich communities, which are becoming greedy and covetous.

From the standpoint of karma it is seen that the world is engulfed by such a disproportionate desire that health is at stake. The half-gained success, the unachieved goals, the hours of exhaustion of soul and body, the emptiness of everything, the months and years of efforts and endeavours, the insuperable odds, the stupendous power of forces, the roaring tide of ignorance are all responsible for the present problems of ill health. This is the global context in which a doctor works on a patient. Medicines alone cannot be an answer; they form a temporary palliation. Excessive medication adds to the problem.

A wise man says one word, "Love! Love perfects all. Let love prevail. Let all men love." This statement seems to be a fallacy, but the magnetism of love entertained in the heart rejuvenates the health and the inner wealth. Love is the reassuring energy that brings in fresh leaves of life. Slowly the medical science will realize the alchemy of thought, and above all, the alchemy of LOVE.

34. Meditation

Meditation has now become a global concept. Many realize that daily meditation helps calming down the system, restoring normalcy of body rhythm. When mind is calmed down it calms down the whole system, the nerves, the circulatory system, the respiratory system, the heart etc. Meditation is a great healing tonic when appropriately used.

There are many significant findings made, working with meditation by various groups. It is also found that meditation helps to reverse some of the ill effects of stress. It can lower the blood pressure, reduce anxiety and anger, relieve from sleeplessness and even from moderate depression.

Scientific experiments are underway regarding changes in the brain when the focus of the mind alters towards sublime thoughts. When man's brain is engaged in sublime thoughts, changes are noticed in the brain. A recent study by US researchers in the universities is revealing answers to the question of what goes on in the brain during meditation. It is observed by such research, which is still in its nebulous state that in people who are stressed, anxious or depressed, the right frontal cortex of the brain is often over-active. And in some cases it is also found that the key brain centre is processing fear. By contrast, it is also observed that people who are usually calm and happy typically show greater activity in the left frontal cortex. They pump out less of stress hormones. It is further observed that there is daily fluctuation of activity between the left and the right frontal cortex brains, depending upon the mood of the people.

The researchers experimented on a group which was divided into meditating and non-meditating people. The meditating group was put to meditation technique for 3 months, gradually increasing the daily time of meditation. After 3 months, when the meditating group was examined with respect to their brains, there was a pronounced shift of activity towards the left frontal cortex. Such a shift did not show in the non-meditators. There was no significant shift. This led to the theory that regular meditation may have shifted the natural 'set point' to the left set point – means, the best point of positioning of man's awareness.

This is a happy and positive note on which further research is proceeding. But from ancient-most times meditation has been seen as 'a wonderful tour' to calm down the brain, which in turn calms down the whole functional system of the human body.

It is time that quietening the mind should be attempted by health workers through conducting meditation camps in serene ambience.

The morning time of dawn and evening hours of dusk are found very appropriate for meditational work. Regular meditation, more or less at the same time, would further help. Meditation after defecation and effective shower with fresh clothing put on has a contributory effect.

Full moon and new moon days are considered much more congenial for good results from meditation. Meditation is, in fact, a way of life whose first impact is on health - a very positive impact.

35. Future School of Medicine

Today, a school of holistic healing is a global thought. Many think of multidisciplinary healing and therapeutic system. A real holistic school of healing is yet to emerge. Experiments are many and all of them are almost partial. It is expected that in this century healers, doctors, psychologists and other health practitioners would open up themselves to constitute a common platform of healing and set the stage for future unfoldment. It is not an easy task, but it is worthwhile to consider a school for such healing technique where growing attitudes towards synthesis are worked out. While such a thought is fraught with many hurdles, progress can nevertheless be made if all participants are willing to lift up their mental barriers. A possible school for such future healing would embody:
- psychological adjustments and healing,
- magnetic healing,
- the best of the allopathic, ayurvedic and homoeopathic techniques with which we must not dispense,

- surgical healing in its modern forms,
- electrotherapeutics,
- water-therapy,
- healing by colour, sound and radiation,
- preventive medicine,
- the essential practice of osteopathy & chiropractic,
- scientific neurology and psychiatry,
- the cure of obsessions and mental diseases,
- the care of the eyes and ears,
- voice culture, which is a definite agency,
- mental and faith healing, and
- soul alignment and contact.

This type of school demands or expects from each of the disciplines somebody who would teach not only theory but also teach out of his practical experience, involving case study. These teachers have to be essentially practitioners in their respective fields and somebody who has gained adequate practical experience. As between them they need to understand each other's disciplines with open mind and also respect where one can supplement the other. They need to feel as one group and one consciousness, dedicated to healing. They need to learn to concede one system to the other where the other system is found more effective and beneficial.

In such a school, the teacher as well as the students need to know that they are living in momentous times, that they are attempting at a very noble task and that their work is a pioneering work. Finally they need to adjust each other's views to accomplish the goal.

Already there is such co-operation taking place between homoeopathy, ayurveda, naturopathy, preventive medicine, psychology, electrotherapy etc., but it is not adequate. The adequacy comes by including as many systems as indicated above with open-mindedness.

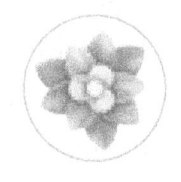

36. Discipleship in Healing

Today there is too much talk on spiritual healing, which seldom happens consciously. Chance healing cannot be ruled out. Such events cannot either be systematized or be claimed as great acts of healing.

Spiritual healing demands many great qualities in a person who is almost saint-like. It is expected that a spiritual healer is in a state of awareness where he is unaffected by the 6 negative qualities, namely:
- excessive desire,
- uncontrollable anger,
- miserly parting with physical objects, emotional and mental thoughts,
- attraction towards worldly things,
- jealously and
- pride.

This state of awareness demands a way of life, which is called discipleship. There is further demand from the spiritual healer of the following qualities:
- harmlessness,
- lack of thieving instinct,

- regulated sex activity,
- alignment between thought, speech and action,
- not getting into obligations by receiving excessive favours from others,
- internal and external purity,
- knowledge of health,
- cheerfulness and humour,
- and above all, that rare quality of LOVE.

The 6 negative qualities transmuted into 6 positive qualities, plus these 8 qualities enable a pure instrument of the healer, that can transmit life energies from the surroundings via himself through the hands, through the looks, through the speech, or through the touch.

Apart from the above, he needs to acquire certain skills, which again are 15 in number. They are as under:
- the skill to contact and work as a soul,
- the skill to command the spiritual will,
- the skill to establish telepathic rapport,
- he must have exact knowledge,
- the skills to reverse, re-orient and exalt,
- the skill to direct the soul's energy to the necessary area,
- the skill to express magnetic purity and the needed radiance,
- the skill to control the activity of the mechanism of the head,

- the skill over his own centres,
- the skill to utilize exoteric and esoteric methods of healing,
- the skill to work magnetically,
- the skill to work with radiation,
- the skill to practise at all times complete harmlessness,
- the skill to control the will and work through love,
- the skill, eventually, to wield the law of life.

Such is the stupendous work to be a true healer.

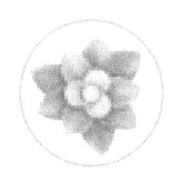

37. Food Subtleties

The modern man gradually realizes that health is directly linked to the nature of his activity, which includes the activity of intake. The modern man also realizes that energy is received not only through food but also through sunlight, air, water, extra-breathing and even through thoughts of goodwill.

Food is not seen as the only source of energy. On the contrary, it is more and more realized that the lesser the calories of food the better is the health and longevity. It is generally known now that green vegetables, leaf vegetables and fruits are the mantrams for longevity. Intelligent and thinking men today prefer raw and fresh vegetables, fruits, juices, much water and sunlight. People prefer high carotene fruits and vegetables to avoid cancer, heart attacks etc. Those who are inclined towards yoga and meditation reduce gradually, but substantially, eating heavy-calorie food, such as meat, roots, specially potatoes, and even pulses and cereals. Sprouted cereals and pulses, salads and raw vegetables replace the heavy food. Studies made in this regard have also proved that the lesser are the calories of food the better is health and longevity.

Many incurable diseases such as diabetes, rheumatic arthritis, obesity, blood pressure, cardiac problems are due to the tendency to eat food of high calories, which is beyond the body's capacity to assimilate. There is a movement emphasizing on the above, besides emphasizing on reducing salt. Salt retains water. The lesser the salt the better is health, says naturopathy and ayurveda.

Many studies have been done with respect to the above, and it is a proven fact.

It is wise to gradually and systematically reduce the calories of food over a couple of years (2 years) than to think of sudden reduction, which would disturb the system.

The medical science needs to recognize that the human bodies are evolving through time and are getting sophisticated and therefore cannot have the same pattern of food as before. The human bodies are not fit anymore for heavy food. Much of the ills today are due to stuffing the body with food that is heavy for the human machine. Indigestion, constipation, accumulation of gases and the consequent sicknesses are due to excessive food consumption. There is definite need to lighten the food. This needs education. The esoteric understanding is that the human brain and human body are evolving every 7 years since World War II – a phenomenon attributed to the New Age planetary energy, Uranus!

Besides, the automation and other mechanical facilities do not let the man of these days to exert physically. Hence he does not burn as many calories as he did before. If man counts the calories that he burns and compares it with the calories of food he eats, he would know how much he overeats. This overeating on the planet is really amazing! It is specially so in the rich communities and developed countries, where the availability of food is very high.

There is every need to balance the daily intake of calories and their expenditure. This knowledge is important, since humans do not physically exert so much, while mentally they do. Mental exertion is subtle exertion and therefore needs subtle food. Subtle food is sunlight, fresh air, water, fruit juices, salads, fresh raw vegetables, but not foodstuffs that are tough for digestion. Man is tending towards a subtle world, and subtle food facilitates the movement into subtle thoughts. Education in this regard needs to happen.

38. Basic Health

Man thinks of health only when he is in disease. He needs to think of health much before. 'Health is wealth', is a known dictum. He should start early in life to give importance to health, as early as seven years of age. The body can be kept hale and healthy if right rhythm, right food and right aspiration are cultivated from childhood.

The wise suggest of instituting health right from the point of impregnation! They advise right attitudes, right food and right activity for the couple who conceives. Right conditions for conception are also recommended. The couple needs to be harmonious and mentally at peace and poise before thinking of conception. They are also required to be healthy physically and emotionally. The time and the place of conception were also given importance.

Likewise there is a discipline throughout pregnancy for the couple to maintain harmony at mind, peace in the emotional plane and health in the body. The mother is advised to follow high standards of food intake, to have regular readings of inspiring lives and wisdom books, to participate in holy congregations and meditation programs. During the first seven months and the next two months a lot can be done to give the right base of health. This base for good health cannot be created later. In fact, wisdom says, a long preparation by the couple before they conceive makes this base even stronger. With basic health if thus made strong as the person grows, one can meet the challenges of the times. 'Basically a healthy person remains healthy even with slight transgression of health rules. Basically an unhealthy person, even if he or she follows the best health regulations, cannot be healthy.' This statement needs to be pondered over.

Conditions at the time of conception, pregnancy and delivery are of paramount importance to provide healthy genes. Any tinkering work to attain health at the later part of life is generally low yielding in results.

One should also note that the soul finds itself in new surroundings at birth and is immersed in a body (the mother), which is at first totally strange to the soul. This loneliness disappears only gradually and can be a source of fear and anxiety. It is therefore all the more necessary to offer congenial and harmonious conditions, lest the soul would be dreaded. The soul also feels imprisoned unless it is well taken care of with knowledge by the couple who conceives.

The young men and women, if well educated on these aspects, can give birth to a healthy race. Instituting health in the prenatal stages is already a great work of healing.

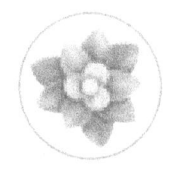

39. Relevance of Astrology

A prophecy was pronounced by a Master of Wisdom during the mid of 20th century that the astrology of the future will indicate the purpose of the soul as distinct from its personality life. This will revolutionize medicine.

It is pertinent to note that the father of the modern medicine, Hippocrates, was considering astrology also as a tool to comprehend the depth and the duration of the sickness. Astrology throws light on the subject of healing. A healer is better equipped if he knows astrology. In all traditional societies the practice of consulting astrologers in matters of health and disease prevails even now. The transit of Saturn, Mars, Moon, Jupiter through various houses and their progression in the personal horoscope are studied in relation to transitory, chronic and sudden acute diseases. The cause for congenital diseases is also seen from the standpoint of karma with the help of astrology. Accordingly the patients psychologically get prepared to accept the duration of sickness. This would lend the cooperation of the patient also for a lengthy treatment.

Though use of astrology for medical purposes is an ancient practice known all over the world, its appropriate and accurate use is generally not. True comprehension of astrology as a science is not yet.

When astrology regains its status of science once again, the charts of the soul and of the personality would be drawn and would be compared. Then by correlation astrological conclusion would be arrived at, and the physician would be on far surer ground than he is now. Till date astrology for medical purposes was used in relation to physical diseases within the physical body. In future it will concentrate upon the condition of the etheric vehicle, which is the transmitter of life energy from the vital body to the physical body of flesh and blood via the glands. This is a new and imminent development in astrological research.

No doubt astrology brings in subjective factors for diagnosis purposes, but it need not be feared as it is not a complicated matter while it appears so to many. When more research and investigation would be carried forward into the future, the science of medicine will be built upon the fact of vital body and its constituent. It will then be discovered that subjective factors of diagnosis are far simpler and less complicated than the present medical science. Today the medicine has reached such a point of complexity that an average medical practitioner cannot cope up with the mass of detailed knowledge now gathered relating to the physical body, its various systems, their interrelation and their effect on many organs, which constitute man. It would therefore eventually need other tools for diagnosis of which astrology would be one.

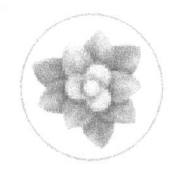

40. Etheric Body (1)

There is an incisive and incessant research to find a medical solution to the present health crises. The new medicine cannot be scientifically formulated and intelligently presented until such time when the fact of etheric body and its existence as a mechanism of energy supply are accepted. There is a subtle mechanism called etheric body that receives the vital solar energy and transmits the same to the physical body. If this body is kept intact, man does not fall sick easily. This body receives and transmits life and light and hence is considered very important in the esoteric circles.

The shift of attention of the medical profession will be then away from the outer, tangible, physical effects to the inner causes. The inner causes will lead the attention to the centres, which are the basis for the glandular functioning.

Within the areas where a disease is manifested, certain esoteric facts anent the general subject are posited hereunder as enumerated by the Tibetan Master:

- That disease in its immediate cause can be traced

to the individual etheric body when the difficulty is purely local or to the planetary etheric body, where epidemics are involved, or to such a condition as war, affecting large masses of men.

- That the etheric body has not hitherto been considered as an existent fact, from the angle of orthodox medicine, though there is a modern drift towards emphasis upon vitality, upon the vital qualities in food and giving of vitamin products in order to build up a vital response. This is the first indication of an unrealized need to increase the potency of the vital body.

- That the condition of the etheric body predisposes the subject to disease or protects it from disease, making man resistant to the impact of the deteriorating or epidemic factors, or failing to do so because of inherent etheric weakness.

- That the etheric body is the mechanism of vital, pranic life and substands or underlies the outer, familiar equipment of the nervous system, which feeds and actuates all parts of the physical organism. The relationship existing between the centres, the nadis and the entire nervous system comprises the field of the new medicine and indicates the new major field of research.

- That the main causes of all disease are two in nature:

1. They are to be found, first of all, in the stimulation or the non-stimulation of the centres. This

stimulation implies the over-activity or the under-activity of any centre in any part of the body. Where the flow of energy is commensurate to the physical body at a particular state of development, there will be relative freedom from disease.

2. They are to be found, secondly, in the karmic effect of the three planetary diseases: cancer, tuberculosis, syphilitic diseases. Some day medicine will realize that behind every single disease (irrespective of the results of accidents or war) lie these three main tendencies in human body. This is a basic and important statement.

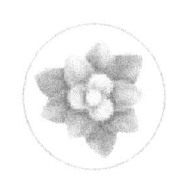

41. Etheric Body (2)

- That the etheric body is a focusing point for all the interior energies of the body, and therefore the energy transmitted will not be pure vital energy or simple planetary prana, but will be qualified by forces coming from the astral or the emotional apparatus, from the mind or from the soul body. These 'qualifications of force' indicating as they do the karma of the individual, are in the last analysis the major conditioning forces. They indicate the point of development of the individual and the areas of control in his personality. They therefore indicate the state of his karma. This lifts the whole subject of medicine into the psychological field and posits the entire problem of karmic effects and ray types.
- That these conditioning factors make the etheric body what it is in any incarnation; these factors are, in their turn, the result of activities initiated and carried through in previous incarnations, and thus constitute the patient's karmic liabilities or his karmic freedoms.
- That the basic energies pouring into the etheric body and conditioning the physical body will be of two

major types: the ray energy of the soul and the ray energy of the personality, qualified by the three minor forces or the rays of the mental nature, the astral body and the physical vehicle. This therefore involves five energies, which are present in the etheric body and which the physician of the future will have to consider.

- That diagnosis, based upon the recognition of these subjective factors, are not in reality the involved and complicated matter they appear to be today to the student of advanced occult theories. Medical men in the New Age will eventually know enough to relate these various ray forces to their appropriate centres. Hence they will know which type of force is responsible for the condition – good or bad – in any particular area of the body. Some day when more research and investigation have been carried forward, the science of medicine will be built upon the face of the vital body and its constituent energies. It will then be discovered that this science will be far simpler and less complicated than the present medical science. Today, medicine has reached such a point of complexity that specialists have perforce been needed who can deal with one area of the body and with its effects upon the entire physical vehicle. The average general practitioner cannot cope with the mass of detailed knowledge now gathered regarding the physical body, its various systems, their interrelations and their effects upon the many organisms which constitute the whole man. Surgery will remain occupied with the anatomical necessities of the human frame. Medicine will shift its focus of attention, before long, to the etheric body and its incident circulatory systems of energy, its interlocking relationships, and the flow between the seven centres, between the centres themselves, and the areas which they control.

This and the previous editorial are an attempt to indicate the lines along which medical research will trend in the next two centuries. The effect of the present day approach to cure sickness here and now will be replaced by a deeper understanding of sickness and the time duration.

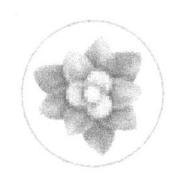

42. Habitation and Health

It was known to Hippocrates, to Paracelsus and such other healers who were more than just physicians that certain lands are healthy and certain lands foster disease and ill health. Dark and crowded tenements, underground houses, flats, moist places where the moist creeps in even through concrete floors, mashie lands are notorious breeding places for disease and ill health.

Not all the underground waters are healthy. All that comes from nature cannot be considered as healthy. Certain waters carry more calcium, certain other waters carry more sulfur. Likewise calcium and other chemicals, iron and other metals exist excessively in waters. In underdeveloped countries people are affected mostly by uncured waters while in developed countries the situation is different.

But in developed countries too the drinking waters have lost much of their health due to an excessive period of storage and sometimes excessive treatments with minerals.

The life that flowing waters carry is different from the life in stored waters. The stagnated waters lose life in them substantially. Water stored in plastic containers is not as healthy as water stored in the earthen pots. The latter enables flow of air through the earthen matter while the former does not enable such flow of life giving air.

While science helps to come out of certain primitive ways of living to bring in health, many of the new measures of handling water bring in new kinds of ill health.

The importance of water is known by all physicians. They should therefore discourage drinking treated water with minerals, stored in plastic containers. Glass containers are considered the best.

In any case the age of the water in the bottle cannot be beyond 7 days from the point of collection for drinking purposes. As much as the quality of water is seen, so much the quality of the water carriers must be seen. A recent study in India revealed that water stored in the brass containers are healthier for drinking purposes, which was a traditional practice now replaced by plastic containers in the urban areas.

The quality of land decides the quality of water and the quality of life. Thus national, regional and rural diseases differ from each other in their causes. Globalization of medicinal standards does not help much in all situations.

Likewise the psychological conditions of a race or a nation have their own tendency to disease. Certain psychologies have lowered resistance to disease while certain other psychologies have better resistance to disease. Some races carry better resistance even to contaminated food and water than certain other races. The immunity system differs from race to race and nation to nation.

The globalization of medicinal standards therefore has to be suitably modified to individual needs of places and groups.

43. Science and Theosophy

Some races are prone to succumb to one form of physical ill while other races are resistant to it. Climatic conditions produce certain types of diseases which are strictly regional. But global diseases such as cancer, heart, brain, syphilis, tuberculosis, psoric diseases, which are rampant are not on the same footing. The global diseases are considered as result of the ignorant life style adopted by humanity in the past. Past does not mean immediate past but remote past such as Atlantean times.

If a global review of health is undertaken, not even a hundred thousand humans could be found perfectly healthy amidst the billions now dwelling on the planet. Frankly speaking, the present medical research and the evolving science of medicine are inadequate to meet the challenge. This gives a dimension: What cannot be cured shall have to be endured. By this approach to life the tension to fight is withdrawn paving way to a better future through endurance of the result of past mistakes. Many times when disease is not given excessive importance and the related attention, it does not grow further, for energy follows thought. This can be further supplemented with the thought of unity, goodwill, love in action besides the science of theosophy.

At present the aforesaid tools are in the hands of devoted but unintelligent people in general. While devotion is desirable, intelligence is equally desirable to bring out the value of these supplementary aids. When the knowledge jealously guarded by these devoted but unintelligent people reaches the hands of the thinkers and the scientists, the many unproved ideas of the former find scientific expression. This would help to reinforce.

The work of psychologists and physicians: When the work of physicians and surgeons in relation to the physical body is recognized as essential and good, when the psychoanalysis and conclusion of the psychologists supplement the work of the physicians and surgeons, and when the power of thought of goodwill and love as coming from theism, likewise aid, then and only then we shall enter upon a new era of well-being.

PS: The thought of goodwill and love include such concepts as yoga, meditation and natural ways of life and thoughts of wisdom.

44. Fourfold Approach

The science of medicine and health would be considered great when the whole man could be healed through bringing together all the available knowledge relating to health and healing, in whatever manner it is presently available. The man's need is holistic health. Such a health has four dimensions: physical, emotional, mental and spiritual. With the available knowledge that man carries in all the four fields, it should not be difficult to attain this. It needs will to join the forces from all four sides.

The physicians and surgeons, the psychologists, neurologists and psychiatrists, the mental healers, new thought workers, and lastly the men of wisdom who know the spiritual dimension of man can bring together their knowledge and practical experience to serve man.

All these four players have their strengths and their limitations. But the limitations of one category can be offset by the strength of the other. They are essentially like the four branches of one tree of health. None of the branches can claim to be the complete tree, however much they claim to be. The human ignorance and the constituent pride are today engaged in a fight as between the four departments, i.e. the physical, emotional, mental and spiritual workers. Each one is claiming to be greater than the other forgetting their complementary nature. The attitude to oppose, discern, disparage and discount the other branches of health science is but ignorance. The time has come and the intelligence of humanity is getting mature demanding openness from all sides. Accommodating others' school of thought to see how it supplements one's own school of thought is emerging in a very small way. It needs to be developed further. This can happen if all health workers at all levels remember that man is more important than their own theories of health and that all that helps to heal man's sickness should be considered as part of the science of health.

45. Homeopathy

Homeopathy was born out of a doctor, a physician, who was an allopath before. It comes through the experiments of Dr. Samuel Hahnemann. It is now disputed in some quarters that if at all homeopathy is a science. Until etheric existence is scientifically acceptable homeopathy cannot be accepted as science. Recently an experiment has been done by Jacques Benveniste and his co-workers, publishing the result of series of experiments on human basophiles. They diluted the basophiles with distilled water to the point where there should have been no antibody molecules left in the solution. But to their surprise they observed a reaction from the basophiles.

Benveniste and his co-workers did further experiments with diluted solutions. To his utter surprise his research showed that even when the allergic substances were further diluted down to homeopathic quantities they could still trigger a reaction in the basophiles!

The basic principle of homeopathy is that a sickness can be cured by small quantities of the substance that has similar qualities as that of the sickness. Now Benveniste's experiment confirms that the water in which a substance is diluted carries the memory relating to the quality of the substance. The quality of the substance is the etheric form of the substance. Thus the etheric, subtle aspect of the substance is given as medicine in homeopathy but not the substance as such. This is where the physicist proclaims that homeo medicine is only sweet pills and has no medicinal substance. It is true that in the dilutions of homeo medicine there is only the memory of the substance but not the substance as such. But now the theory that water carries memory would unfold one more step to accept the science of homeopathy.

In the east it was easy to accept homeopathy due to the oriental belief system which accepts the subtle aspects of a substance as well as the gross aspect of a substance. The homeopaths know for sure that in due course of time the science of homeo would not only become acceptable but would also open doors to cure many emotional and psychic disorders.

Time proves the science of every fiction.

46. Sickness – the Doorway to Health

Sickness many times leads to better health and even longevity. This looks to be a fallacy, but it is true. For example when man finds himself slightly diabetic he takes to better routine, with choicest food, exercise etc. What is not possible in healthy condition sometimes becomes possible when there is ill health. The fear of ill health would many times work out to be attentive in matters of health habits. Until man really evolves he would not be self-responsible in matters of health. Majority of mankind still remains in infancy or adolescence. They are yet to be self-responsible. People that are mature are conscious of the consequences of their actions. Such people implicitly take to daily exercise, right food, right action, right thought and adequate sleep. The ones who do not take to this discipline are disciplined by nature by throwing signals of danger in matter of health.

Diabetes, cardiac problems or hypertension drive patients to right discipline. When the related discipline is implemented they live longer than many. They take to a new rhythm and place themselves in a new life pattern.

The patients who know their sickness most and who take to the right discipline are the ones that live the longest.

Regular and brisk physical activity, which is frequently emphasized, is the greatest causality of a healthy life amidst the humans. In all sick people one generally finds aversion to physical activity. Out of fear the ones that fall into sickness, get into exercise at doctor's advice and take to a healthy life style. That is how most of the sick who take to the discipline inevitably fall into the slot of healthy life style. They live long by adopting to the healthy rhythm.

Likewise people susceptible to heart disease, blood pressure etc., who notice their sickness in the early stages maintain better health due to the early advise they receive to prevent sickness. This is because they respond out of concern to the meaningfulness of right food, right exercise, relaxed attitude to work and good sleep.

Even the most educated in the society are very poor in their attitude to health until they are hit hard, but sometimes it could be too late. The rich are as poor in their knowledge as the uneducated, considering the oily foods, the sweets, the ice creams and other high calorie food they eat.

Education relating to the life style is a much more valuable service to health than treating the sickness. There has to be as much education of health as medication at the least.

47. Vaccines

There are age old misgivings about inoculation and vaccination. This question is often in the minds of healers and health practitioners. They feel that inoculation and vaccination affect the subtle bodies. This is not true. The science of inoculation is purely physical in origin. There is no occult standard or value in inoculation. The entire question concerning serums and inoculation has been tremendously over-emphasized by the so-called healers and health workers. They do not understand that the human body in the present times is recipient of many and varied extraneous substances from the ever deteriorating environment. The whole subject has a vaster import than what people think of. There are greater dangers to which man's body is presently exposed than the exposure to vaccinations. People are generally blissful of impending dangers and worry over trivials. "When the whole city was burning a woman was crying for having burnt the frills of the frock."

Wrong food of every kind, inhalation of smoke from centuries, breathing in polluted air, taking poisonous medicines, pills, and tablets, injections of mineral substances, of drugs and serums into the human body have vaster import than inoculation and vaccinations. The remarkable assimilative powers of the human body are a wonder. Hence the concern over inoculation and vaccinations is misplaced.

On the contrary it should be said in all fairness that as far as the physical well-being of man is concerned the techniques and methods developed by the West resulted in a healthier race in the West than in the East, in prolonging human life and eliminating dire physical scourges.

The effect on the inner bodies is practically nil and far less than the diseases which are prevented through vaccination. The science of inoculation and vaccinations is purely physical in origin and concerns only the physical part of the body. It does not affect the emotional or mental body.

The only part relating to this science which is of concern is that to control diseases in man, the substance taken from the bodies of the animals is injected into human body. Science will have to supersede this by a higher technique. Until such time the available remedies cannot be thrown out. Commonsense and science should overcome the superstitious beliefs.

48. Earth – Health

The atomic structures of all forms including the physical body of man are based on the atomic structures of the Earth preserved over millions of years. The spirit of Earth preserves its hold upon such structures. During the incarnated experience of any soul the elements of Earth were temporarily isolated from Earth. It gathers together again the elements of its like and reabsorbs those elements into itself. Earth gives forms and takes them away which is seen as incarnation and dis-incarnation of the soul.

These atoms, it must be noted, are conditioned by two factors, for which the spirit of Earth is solely responsible: firstly the karma of the planet, secondly the limitation of physical plane matter of the Earth. The matter of the planet is evolutionary in nature. The soul that incarnates is evolving too.

Besides the elements of the planet itself are under evolution. They have their own imperfection. They too contribute to the diseases. It is for this reason the planet is not considered perfect.

The point in evolution of the spirit of Earth affects every atom in the bodies produced from it. The result of this imperfection of the Earth shows itself in the presence of disease in all forms and in all kingdoms of nature. Minerals are subject of disease and decay. Metals too have their 'fatigue'. Plants and animals react to disease within the structure of the form. Thus disease and death are inherent in the very atom of which all organisms are composed. Man is not exempt from this general condition.

Often attributing disease to the wrong thinking of man is not entirely true. This is inherent in the form coming from Earth.

It is therefore all the more necessary that we do not spoil what is already there in nature by our irresponsibility. The nature of the planet is inherently sick. We cannot by our irresponsibility contribute to further sickness.

This dimension of Earth and its inherent imperfection should be given due consideration. Man incarnates into such substance and form, which has conditioning and limitation. With his awareness and relative perfection he should assist but not destroy the elements. He should assist for its progress. His progress is inbuilt in the progress of the atomic substance of Earth. He should assume responsibility for the progress of the elemental form. This is where man has a great divine responsibility.

49. The Man – His Humous Form

It is a generally known factor in the wisdom circles that man develops the earthy vehicle around him, which is called the human body. He incarnates and gathers around him the form, which is composed of substance of the Earth, which is already subjected to the conditioning. The substance he gathers around him into his form is the substance of this Earth, which has its limitations. The form is humous, i.e of Earth. The man is the dweller. Humous and man constitute hu-man, human. The planet Earth is upon the evolutionary arch and has therefore its imperfections. Its matter is subject to karma. It has its limitations. They affect the physical form composed of such substance. The incarnating soul (the man) acquires an imperfect form, which has its inherent limitations and the related sicknesses. The form thus acquired is partially useful to him and is partially troublesome also. In the initial years (up to 35 years) it grows and cooperates. In the later 30 years its cooperation generally comes down and later limits the dweller of the body.

It should be understood that as much the indweller receives help from the form he also helps the substance of the form contributing to its evolution. This is where responsibility is cast on man to improve the quality of substance on the planet starting with the substance of his body and the bodies that he performs to his progeny. This in turn improves the quality of form he receives.

'The will to live' is the greatest factor in man's life that generally decides his longevity in the form. However much the form makes man suffer, the will to live anchors him to the form. This will to live also needs to be examined with respect to the patients in cases of fatal sicknesses. If there is strong will to live, he can survive even from fatal, advanced sickness. The power of the soul transmits the related life energies through will.

Doctors would do well to encourage this will in the patients through positive (yet not false) approach.

It is said from ancient most times, "Where there is will, there is way." It should also be known in this context that it is the will of the soul to live that is important, but not the wish of the mind (personality).

The will of the soul enables the incarnation of the soul. It does so for reasons of purpose. The purpose of the soul has to be fulfilled in the journey of life. Normally as man grows the purpose is forgotten and man estranges himself into pleasures of life. If the purpose is not pursued a mere wish of the mind to live will not help.

Great beings who lived for noble purposes could continue to live longer in spite of a disabled body. Some could depart very early when their purpose was fulfilled. It is therefore important to see the purpose of life from the standpoint of the soul to prolong the life in the body. This is also important from the healing angle.

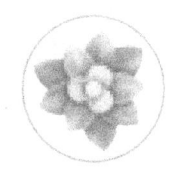

50. A Prophecy

"As a few decades elapse there would be a happy union between the medical profession and healers with true spiritual perception. The medical science will find simple ways of treatment, which are nearer to the laws of nature," says a seer.

In the medical profession there are, here and there, true thinkers who look for more satisfying solutions to restore health than what exists today. From out of them, it is possible that trendsetters could be born like Paracelsus, Hahnemann, Kent etc. These thinkers are growing in number due to the dissatisfaction they experience in the wild jungle of antibiotics, cortisones, sleeping pills, pain killers, radiations, chemotherapies etc.

They cannot as yet embrace the so-called spiritual healers whose weaknesses and limitations are too many. These thinkers would grow out of the genuine need they feel for true treatment of the patients. When the feeling grows deeper and touches their heart, they would intuitionally perceive certain dimensions called 'spiritual', which would incline them to look fresh at the esoteric teachings on health and healing. Since their search is with a scientific approach, they find the truth of spiritual laws, one by one. Their understanding of these laws would be more balanced and less emotional. What little they perceive would be far more true to them than what a faith based healer says. But as the physician progresses he finds the hidden science in the faith claims of spiritual healers.

This apart, more and more men and women of spiritual orientation will enter the medical profession and gradually perfect themselves in the techniques of orthodox medicine and in the exoteric knowledge of anatomy and pathology. They would further equip themselves with the remedies as are available. They would add their understanding and knowledge coming from esoteric learning and combine with the growing numbers of true thinkers that are in pursuit of holistic healing.

In the meanwhile the healers can take to the learning of physical anatomy and pathology and the physicians can learn the occult anatomy as well as the pranic pulsations and glandular functions as given in the esoteric literature.

Open-minded thinkers are growing in both the fields, which would enable dispassionate consideration of each other's claims. Repudiating the claims of each other is infancy. Considering the truth of the claims with a gentle attitude is maturity.

The sincerity of majority of those who belong to different schools of thought is unquestioned, but at the same time there are also charlatans to be found in a very small way. These are generally self-seeking ignorant exploiters. They are in general commercially oriented. This minority section generally controls and limits the majority. This is the case in all walks of life. A selfish, non progressive minority limits and controls the majority. Nevertheless sincere investigators and lovers of humanity in both the groups are the future hope of the medical science. The need of humanity would bring about the desired orientation in all the different schools of thought relating to the medicine. The physicians would commute to bring the gift of new era healing.

51. Post Death Healing

Be it healers or doctors, all meet their helplessness in healing when a patient approaches death. They may even entertain a sense of futility. They feel that their efforts have terminated into a stunning disability. In spite of all their knowledge and their will to aid to restore the departing one, there seems nothing to be done but to step aside with a sense of futility while the patient is passing through the exit gates of life to the in-gates of death.

Nowadays there is increased belief even in the West that the soul survives and reincarnates. Even this deep-seated belief in the persistence of the immortal soul proves inadequate. The serving healer may at best console himself with this belief. Nevertheless at the back of his mind he feels his limitation.

But the healer and the doctor can help further, though not for restoration of life but for peaceful and comfortable departure of the soul into the subtle world. This knowledge and practice of such knowledge is part of healing, many times a very effective practice.

There is as much healing that can be offered to the patient after death, as it is done before death. But this part of healing is to be done more by the family of the departed person. The healing work after death can be briefly stated as under:

- maintaining serene, silent, and peaceful atmosphere with light music (violin) in the background, in the room where the body is kept,

- lighting sandal wood incense in the room where the body is kept before its cremation or burial,

- placing a lighted lamp behind the head till the body is moved to the burial or cremation ground,

- taking home and retaining the body at home for the near and the dear to pay homage is far better than taking the body to burial ground straight away from the hospital where the patient died.

The esoteric wisdom enunciates that the departed soul hovers around the dead body till it is cremated or buried. Hence any acts of goodwill done before the burial are very helpful to the soul in its journey. Normally such acts are done within 10 days from the date of departure. Reading scriptures relating to the immortality of the soul and guiding the soul into the realms of light is also helpful. Chanting mantras is also done in the East.

In the times to come, this practice of post death healing would be better understood and practiced than now. When man knows that he comes back to fulfill the unfulfilled aspects of life, death would be observed more as a facility to change over into a fresh body, a more sophisticated equipment, from the present decaying and disabled body. Resistance to death would then no more be.

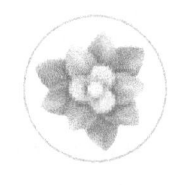

52. 3 + 5 = 8 and 9

Esoterically man is understood as soul. He has a triple capacity emanating from him as will, knowledge, and action. This is called the triad. To manifest the will with the help of knowledge as action he also has a fivefold body, which is constituted of 5 elements, 5 pulsations, 5 sensations, 5 senses and 5 limbs of the body.

He is one and he has 3 and 5 with him. Health or ill health depends upon how the 8 are put to use by man. Many times they use the man instead of man using them. The 8 constitute the form of man and man is the 9th one. When the man, the soul, controls the form, there is health. If not, there is ill health. This is the esoteric understanding of health.

Man is the builder of his form. He supplies forces to the form. He needs to know how to use this form, just like a driver of an automobile needs to know how to drive the automobile. If he does not know, he causes accidents. So is the case with man who does not know his form. He should know his form and its potential. He should also know the nature of his form and the forces that are working in the form. He should use them appropriately. He needs to learn how to apply his will and his knowledge, how to act, when to act, how not to act, when not to act. Wholeness in thought, right relation, goodwill in activity are therefore recommended by the knowers of all times.

The soul is the major energy centre that controls the body and when the soul controls the body man remains the master. This mastery can be gained over the form through experience but not through suppression of the natural appetites of body and mind. Religions that indoctrinate suppression also contributed to ill health, while licenses caused rampage of ill health.

Through experience the soul gradually gains the ability to control the forces of the form nature. The ability to overcome ill health is basically dependent upon the individual experience and the related knowledge gained by each soul.

Mankind as a whole is making a great adventure on the planet. It is also seen as advancement. Each one is at different level of experience and hence all men have different exposures to ill health depending upon their evolution. The healers and doctors would therefore do well to have an insight of the patient's maturity as soul and his attitudes and aptitudes towards the form nature. The culture, tradition and the way of life of a patient would throw greater insight relating to the maturity of the patient. This is where a family doctor who knows the family for generations is preferable to a totally strange and unknown physician. In this world of commercial medicinal activity there is thus reappearance of the need for personalized healing and medical treatment.

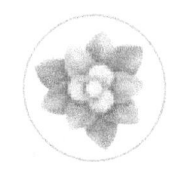

53. Doing – Being

The sick need to be educated. It is also part of healing. Many times right education of health and healing help not only prevention of sickness but cure as well.

Many sicknesses emerge from man's desires, ambitions, and selfish attitude. From the worldly standpoint ambition helps personal growth. Desires fulfill man's longings and selfishness is also seen as self-preservation. But over-ambition, utter selfishness and excessively indulgent desire can and would disturb health. The sick should know this. They are causing disturbance to their health due to their own orientation towards life.

In the present day context of excessive competition, expansionism and covetous feeling, there is an upsurge of anxiety, fear and tension disturbing the solar plexus centre. Once this centre is disturbed man opens the door for sickness. If the aforesaid anxiety, fear etc. continue to exist they cause pressure on pancreas, liver and stomach. Once these organs are affected by continuous pressure they would disturb the whole system including the digestive system, defective system, respiratory system and circulatory system. Anxiety and fear when entertained for long years would bring in hypertension, high blood pressure, production of gases in stomach, sleeplessness and even depression. The area below the diaphragm in the body is the birth place of all sicknesses and hence it cannot be neglected at any cost. But it is put to disturbance through man's incorrect orientation towards life.

Man has been hunting for fulfillment of desires ever since the time of Atlanteans and it is a never ending process. He needs to look back and see if his will to grow is all that worthy resulting in sacrifice of health. He should ask himself if money, power and position are worthier than his own health and well-being. In the East there is a saying, "It is worth drinking a glass of cool water than running for an evasive milk can." The anxiety in running for milk disturbs the system while a glass of cool water taken with quiet mind can nourish the system. Man's relentless hunt for objective expansion is reaching disproportionate heights with devastating consequences in his health system.

There is a story in Upanishads relating to man, who endlessly strives for power and money. He is compared to a jackal who finds a blood stained sword left out by a hunter. The jackal licked the blood stains left over the sword. As he licked he found more and more blood coming through the sword. He licked and further licked the sword until he died. Likewise man today runs crazy after his unfulfilled ambitions and desires, least understanding that his crazy activity is self-destructive. It is evident that the sword does not yield blood, yet the jackal went on pursuing, drinking its own blood which emerged from its licking the sword. Likewise man conditioned by 'will to money' and 'will to power' is running crazily exhausting his own energies.

The seers in the East say the 'will to be' is healthy. The 'will to power and money' can disturb the equilibrium of health. 'To be and to do' is better than only 'to do with disregard to be-ness'. Be-ness is the base. Doing is a dance on that base. If there is no base or insecure base the doing is bound to be affected and in turn affects the doer.

It's about time that man learns to balance his excessive doings and finds equilibrium. Excessive dynamism burns up. The dynamism has to be tempered with static dynamism.

54. Karma and Health

The ancients spoke about 'liberation'. The moderns speak of 'liberty'. Liberty is seen as freedom from any imposition of rule, freedom to do as one wishes, freedom to think and to live as one chooses. This freedom or liberty is sensible when man also accepts responsibility. Today for many moderns, freedom or liberty means freedom without responsibility. They would not like to be responsible for the wishes they fulfill, choices they make, and thoughts that they entertain. Such freedom is nothing but selfishness coupled with ignorance. Freedom or liberty doesn't go hand in hand with selfishness. As a consequence the wrongly understood freedom led many to illnesses besides varieties of conditioning. The ignorance that these liberty lovers carry disables them to see the consequence of their desires, choices and thoughts. Diseases breed from irresponsible acts of indulgences, emotions, and thoughts of selfish nature.

Man is as yet not free from selfish desire and his selfishness motors him to do acts which would be painful to the surrounding life. His attitude towards nature and life carries much ignorance in it. Man continuously hurts the other kingdoms of nature and is hence hurt in turn. He is unconscious that he hurts the animal kingdom, the plant kingdom and the mineral kingdom. He also hurts the intelligences relating to water, i.e. the rivers and oceans. Man cannot escape the consequences of his acts, which boomerang on him in turn. He is promoting the activity of hurt on one side and attending to his own sickness on the other side. He least realizes that the law of karma is inescapable. The situation of man is like a biting dog that bites. He receives bites and keeps licking his own wounds. This may look derogatory or degrading, but this message may be taken positively. Today the nations are reaping what they sowed by way of diseases, calamities, crises one after the other.

This great law of karma is now a recognized factor in human thinking. The question 'why' so frequently asked by man, brings in the concept of causes and effects with constant inevitability. The concepts of heredity, of environment, of placement in life, racial characteristics, local and nations' temperaments, historical causes, social superstitions, blind religious beliefs are all seen from the standpoint of karma.

The law of karma informs every person what health or ill health he brought with him from previous lives and how he should progress to improve health and gradually eliminate the ill health. Liberation of the ancients was a process of liberating oneself from selfish desires, choices and thoughts. In that process, liberation from ill health was also seen. This is where karmic liabilities find a place for consideration by the healer when he proposes to heal a sick person. Just medicines or healing techniques do not cure sicknesses until the karma is experienced and is thus neutralized.

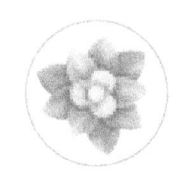

55. Knowledge and Health

The physicians deal with glands, the healers deal with centres. The glandular functioning is connected with the personality of man. The personality cannot change through medicine. It can be changed only through certain self-imposed disciplines which are generally called 'yoga disciplines' or 'the disciplines for the disciples'. It is fundamentally impossible to change the personality and the physical equipment through treating the glands. On the contrary, the glands change when the personality changes through disciplines.

It is generally believed that the physical body is a conditioning body and that man suffers from its conditioning. Even the religions preach that it is sinful to be in the physical body which conditions the man, the soul. The body of flesh and blood is seen even as a sin pot by the religionists. This is ignorance. The physical body is a victim of man's personality. It is the personality life of man that generates forces which are routed through the centres and glands. If the personality is an integrated one, harmonious energy generates and flows through the centres, glands, the endocrine system etc., causing no disturbance to the body. But if the forces generated are of emotional or conflicting nature, they also flow through centres disturbing the centres. When the centres are disturbed the glands are disturbed and consequently irregular secretions happen, causing sickness in the body.

More than with physiology the medical profession needs to engage with the science of psychology. Unless man knows the consequences of the conflicting forces that he engages with and entertains in him, he would not give weightiness to the values of life. The values of life are time-tested ones. They are practiced not just for being accepted as a good person but for establishing harmony within. Where there is inner harmony, there is greater possibility of health. If there is emotional and mental turmoil, such turmoil disturbs the etheric web and affects the physical body.

The quality of the personality again depends upon the point of evolution reached by man. Hence in the process of evolution through trial and error man learns to hold better health through values which are natural and normal. Difficulties do arise in the individuals as long as there is the conflict of what he considers good and bad and the conflict of the pairs of opposites. Thus health is seen as a co-existing factor with knowledge. As knowledge grows in practice, ill health reduces. The knowledge spoken of here is the knowledge of neutralizing the conflicting forces of emotions, thoughts and pairs of opposites. Thus knowledge is the antidote against sickness.

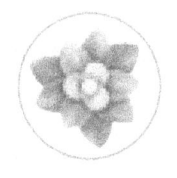

56. The Significant Shift

The inflow of prana, its reception by the etheric body and transmission by the etheric centres of the body gives clues for a fuller comprehension of the laws of health. The health in the physical body depends upon the unimpeded flow of life and this flow of life in the body corporeal happens through the cooperative action of the atoms of the physical body of man. The cooperative action between the etheric body and the physical body and the effective functioning of the etheric body as a receptor and transmitter of prana, shall be the future study relating to health.

It is commonly known that the sunrays carry the life energies and these rays, in interaction with the air around earth, cause golden hue pranic emanations, which are received by the beings on the planet. These golden hue rays conserve the bodies of the beings, preserving the health. It is for this reason the sun is seen as preserver of life.

There are of course other rays coming from the sun, which act differently to cause destruction. We are here concerned with the pranic solar emanations, which are generally available during the dawn and the dusk hours. They are the basis of all physical plane life.

The etheric body is a network, like that of a web, permeated with fire and is animated by the golden light stated above. This golden etheric web is frequently described as the golden bowl in the theologies. The denser matter of the physical plane coheres to the vitalized form of the golden web and builds itself around the web forming into one unit. This web receives life force (prana) and distributes it to the physical body.

Spleen is the organ of reception in the physical body. It receives the prana distributed by its etheric counterpart. It distributes such prana to the base centre, from where prana gets distributed over the entire body and even shines forth beyond the surface of the body as the pranic aura. The spleen is as yet little known in the medical science as to its complete potential. In the study of prana and health of the physical body, functioning of the spleen has a vital role to play.

Likewise the etheric web of the human body, which stands immediately behind the physical body, needs to be understood as more real than the physical body. Its functioning leads to the better understanding of the mechanism of prana working through the human system.

The medical science is beginning to study 'the vitality factor' as the effect of solar rays upon the physical organism. The scientists are trying to study the laws of the radiatory heat within the form. They are able to link up the functions of the spleen to the effect of the action of the glands and their relation to assimilate the vital essence of the bodily frame. As they proceed in these lines, it is most likely that they touch upon the fact of the etheric body. When the basic functions of the etheric body are established, the work of preventive and curative medicine will shift its emphasis to higher levels. The laws of health stand revealed, which can be gained fully steered for the benefit of humanity. This would be a significant shift in the field of health where the focus is more on the etheric body than on the physical automaton.

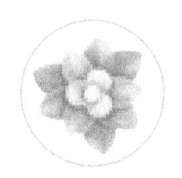

57. Threefold Pranic Supply

Prana is supplied to human forms in three ways. They can be called as solar prana, planetary prana and prana of the pranic forms of earth. They are also respectively termed as golden prana, violet prana and pale violet or grey prana. This is an esoteric understanding.

Solar prana: It is the vital and magnetic fluid that radiates from the sun, which is transmitted to man's etheric body through the agency of certain intelligences of air. These are called in the occult circles as the devas of the golden hue. This prana is of a very high order, which is passed through the airy devas of dolden hue. The powerful golden hue radiations are received at certain etheric centres of the human body: in the forehead and in the shoulder blades. From these etheric centres, this prana gets transmitted down to the physical organ, the spleen.

The golden hued pranic entities are in the air above us and are especially active in the tropical countries, where the air is pure and dry. California is considered to be one such tropical area, where this golden hue is tangible. The rays of the sun in the tropics are considered to be especially beneficial. The tropical belt is the belt of abundant light.

The relation between man and the group of devas mentioned above is very close. Hence the interaction has to be appropriate. Excessive interaction with these rays can cause the menace of sunstroke.

When the medical science comprehends the functioning of the etheric body and its assimilative functions, man can grow immune to the dangers of solar radiations. These deva entities of golden hue are considered as male-female in the occult science. They are females in relation to their ability to receive from the sunrays the vital and magnetic fluid of prana. They are male in relation to distribution of the pranic energies to man and to others forms of life on earth.

It is for this reason, intelligent exposure to the golden light of the sun during the morning and evening hours was considered to be a healthy practice by the ancients of the tropics. It is for the same reason that they clothed the upper parts of the body scarcely compared to the body below navel.

Planetary prana: This is the pranic force emanating from the planet. This pranic force is nothing but the golden hue prana received by the planet from the sun and radiated through its surface. This is an indirect prana, which has undergone certain processes and therefore carries the colour and quality of the planet. The planet absorbs solar prana, assimilates what is required for it and radiates the surplus, which is called planetary radiation. This planetary emanative prana is qualitative and is transmitted by certain intelligences, the devas of air, which are called the devas of violet hue. This prana carries the magnetism of earth, which helps the forms on earth at a lesser level.

The prana of forms: This is the third category of prana available on earth, which is again the pranic radiation from all forms of earth such as plant, animal and humans. These emanations from the beings of earth are ranked third and their impact also exists around. They are of a lesser order and are almost considered as carrying the energies of pale violet or grey.

58. Upset and Set Up

When man understands the threefold prana supply to him – namely from the sun, from the planet and from the forms of life on earth – and when he understands that the three pranic emanations are rated differently, he should be wise enough to choose the best of the prana supply in preference to the 2nd and 3rd grade prana. His preferences also have to be in the same order.

Solar prana transmitted by the airy devas as golden hue during morning and evening hours is by far the best prana, which can be received through exposure to the morning and evening sunrays and also through intense breathing exercises during morning and evening hours.

The ancients knew this. They therefore preferred morning and evening times as the best times for health practices. Exposing to the morning and evening rays and breathing to the lungs capacity during the two times was a common practice. The Greeks and the Romans too knew this like in the East. Games were organised only in these hours with shoulder blades and spleen exposed to sunrays. Breathing fresh air and exposing to sunrays was seen as essential part of life.

The modern life is tending gradually away from this healthy, natural system. Many of the houses that are built today, specially in crowded places, neither receive the golden light of the sunrays nor allow free flow of breeze through the houses. Furthermore houses are built in such a manner that lighting is found necessary even during daytime. There are rooms and chambers in the houses, which never see the daylight nor do they receive breeze. Cross ventilation for free passage of air, adequate windows for the free entry of sunrays seldom happen. In the name of comfort people build close houses where heating or cooling is artificially arranged. Consequently the immune system has become weak in the present times.

The ancient civilizations were all built not on the seashores as today, but on the riverbanks. Ganges and Indus in India, Nile and Jordan in the Middle East, Rhine and Rhone in Europe, Mississippi and Missouri in North America, Amazon in South America are but a few examples. The ancients were building civilizations in riversides, the reason being availability in abundance of the five elements of nature. They never considered the seashore healthy, for seawaters are not healthy waters. They are salty and medicinal. Taking daily baths in rivers was considered healthier, because they were drinkable and life-giving waters. Seawaters were occasionally used on astrologically important days. London, Paris, Brussels, Berlin, Rome, Madrid, Athens, Constantinople, Jerusalem, Delhi, Mexico City are but few examples of ancient cities, none of which was built on the sea shore. It is global business considerations that gave birth to cities on the seashore, where the natural conditions of health are not the same as in other places.

With the sky rise buildings and crowded buildings and with mitigated exposure to golden hue rays, humanity is today dependent more on planetary prana than on solar prana. Secondary prana is in primary use, while primary prana is relegated to background. Added to this, the 3rd grade prana emitted in the crowded places from the co-human beings is getting dominant. The planetary prana and its emanations, which are abundantly available in nature is kept at a distance. The modern man thus is tending towards the 3rd grade prana. Furthermore he brings into the dwelling places where he lives, the domesticated animals such as cats and dogs. He lives with them and sleeps with them.

To such ignorance man is tending in the name of modern life. To him medicines are of no avail. Man should learn to reverse this order. He should set up the right order in this upset situation.

59. The Fires in the Body

"Sickness is unknown to the man, who absorbs and distributes prana (life force) with accuracy", says the occult science. All physicians, health and healing workers need to ponder upon this. When the above statement is properly comprehended, there would be a basic change in the approach of medicine for curative and preventive treatments.

To comprehend the above statement, the working of various fires within the body has to be understood. While prana is seen as active radiatory heat and fire received from the sun and from the planet, the human bodies consist of innumerable cells, wherein there is the latent heat and fire. The active radiatory fire when it finds its blending with the latent fire of the cells of the body, health gets established. The latent fire is the basis of life while the active fire is the stimulator and animator of such life. The latent fire is life of the spheroidal cell or atom. Life moves in these cells as heat with rotary motion. The active fire, prana, is the driving force of the cell forms of the body. It animates the body and even evolves the form. It is in this body of double fire, man exists with the fire of mind. The pranic fire and the cell fire are in constant interaction causing the development of the matter of the body by means of friction. When much prana is invoked, received and distributed thoroughly in the system, the impurities in the cells of the body are cleansed due to the interaction between the latent heat of the cell and the active heat of the prana. The latent heat in the cell is fire imprisoned by the surrounding matter. When it receives external support, it gains the related strength to break through the inertia of matter. Just like the chick in the egg breaks through the shell to grow, when it receives additional heat from the hen. Pranic fire is like the hen and cell fire is like the chick. The former needs to support the latter for growth and for health.

In the physical body, these fires are centralised at the base of the spine. They are situated at a spot at the tip of the spine. This spot of heat radiates in all directions using the spinal column as a channel. It has a special connection to the spleen, the latter being the supplier of the pranic fire. Thus the proper functioning of spine and spleen are of great importance for the physical well-being of man. When the spine is free from the congestion that it suffers and when the spinal column is duly adjusted and aligned, there would be free flow and blending of the two fires, which results in a healthy condition. In such cases the dense physical body would suffer little troubles.

A Master of wisdom compares the spot of the spine to a burning furnace and pranic fire as fuel to keep the fire burning in the furnace. Appropriate supply of fuel would keep the furnace ablaze. The secret to health is thus seen in the occult science as the blending of the active fire and the latent fire. This is the area where the science and occult science could meet to find solutions to sickness.

60. Prana – Reception, Assimilation and Circulation

The ABC of bodily health is wrapped up in the right reception of prana, its assimilation and distribution to the physical body. Man has to make basic changes to ensure these three aspects of the work of prana. The centres whereby the reception of prana is brought about must be allowed to function without impediment.

Pranic emanations from the sun are absorbed by the etheric centres, which are found principally in the upper part of the body, such as the forehead, the shoulder blades and the centre above the diaphragm. From these centres they are directed to the etheric spleen and from the etheric spleen to the spleen of the physical body. The main centre for the reception of prana at present is the centre between the shoulder blades. Other centres of reception are dormant, owing to centuries of wrong living and basic mistakes in relation to natural way of life. The three pranic centres of reception are not in good working order. Only the centre between the shoulder blades is in best receptive condition. Even this receptivity is disturbed, owing to poor condition of the spinal column. In most of the cases, the alignment of the spinal column is not accurate and is slightly misplaced. While the receptive centres of prana are thus functioning in the sub-normal level, the spleen of man is also not adequately developed. Its size today is sub-normal and its vibration is not considered adequate in the esoteric circles.

Where the life is led more normally and naturally, where the upper part of the physical body is adequately exposed to the golden rays of dawn and dusk sun and where man is not a slave of physical comforts, there better conditions are found for reception and assimilation of prana. The aboriginal dwellers seem to carry more effective etheric centres than the civilised man. The civilised man's life conditions are far from natural and normal.

In the coming times, the necessity of exposing the centre between the shoulder blades and the centre above the diaphragm to the rays of the sun will be more appreciated. This exposure improves the physical vitality and makes man adaptable to the changing weathers.

It must be remembered that reception of prana is to enable such prana to interact with the latent heat existing in the physical body cells. When prana functions through the etheric centres adequately, it cooperates with the natural latent bodily warmth, holding the body in a vitalised condition. It imposes upon the matter of the body, giving the required rate of vibration, leading to the healthy functioning of the body organs.

The pranic heat purifies the cell matter, reduces their density, enabling healthy contact between the latent heat of the cell matter and the active heat of prana. Yoga asanas, exercises, breathing practices, physical exertions – they all help in this direction. They would keep the body agile, active and healthy. Bodily inertia should therefore be seen by a physician as inactive functioning of the two fires within.

When prana is received by the two etheric centres (the centre between the shoulder blades and the centre above the diaphragm) and distributed to the etheric counterpart of spleen, then the three centres form into a triangle. The pranic fire circulates thrice through this triangle and is supplied thereafter to the physical organ of the spleen. Thereafter the physical prana is transmitted to the base of the spine to link up to the latent heat of the body. When such link up happens adequately, the fire of prana and the heat of the body cure and provide a very healthy condition to man.

This understanding of the occult science could be helpful to open-minded physicians, healers and health workers.

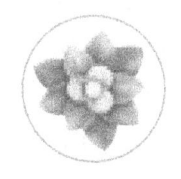

Other Books & Booklets* through the Pen of Dr. Sri K. Parvathi Kumar

The following books are available in:
English (E), German (G), Spanish (S), French (F), Hebrew (H), Telugu (T), Hindi (HI) and Kannada (K) languages.

1. Agni. . . . . E/G/S
2. Amanaskudu . . . . T/K
3. Antardarsana Dhyanamulu . . . . T
4. Anveshakudu . . . . T
5. Asangudu . . . . T
6. Ashram Leaves . . . . E/G/S
7. Ayurvedic Principles. . . . . E
8. Bharateeya Sampradayamu . . . . T
9. Bhriktarahitatarakarajayogamu * . . . . . T/K
10. Dhanakamuni Katha. . . . . T
11. Doctrine of Eternal Presence . . . . E
12. Gayatri Mantra Avagahana . . . . T
13. Geetopanishad – Gnana Yogamu . . . . . T

14. Geetopanishad – Karma Yogamu . . . . . . T
15. Geetopanishad – Sankhya Yogamu . . . . . T
16. Good Friday * . . . . E/G/S/F/HI
17. Guru Paduka Stawam . . . . T
18. Hercules – The Man and the Symbol . . E/G/S
19. Himalaya Guru Parampara (The Hierarchy) * T /HI
20. Indian Tradition * . . . . T
21. Jupiter – The Path of Expansion . . . . E/G/S
22. Jyotirlinga Yatra . . . . T
23. Karma Sanviasa Yoga. . . . . T
24. Karma Yoga . . . . T
25. Katha Deepika . . . . T
26. Listening to the Invisible Master * . . E/G/S/F/H
27. Lord Maitreya – The World Teacher * . . E/G/S/F
28. Mana Master Garu . . . . T
29. Mantrams – Their Significance and Practice E/G/S
30. Maria Magdalena * . . . . E/S
31. Marriage – A Sacrament * . . . . E
32. Master C.V.V. – Yogamu - Karma Rahityamu . . T
33. Master C.V.V. – Yogamu . . . . T
34. Master C.V.V. – The Initiator, Master E.K. – The Inspiror T
35. Master C.V.V. – May Call! . . . . . . E/G/S
36. Master C.V.V. – May Call! II . . . . . . E
37. Master C.V.V. (Birthday Message) * . . . . . T
38. Master E.K. – The New Age Teacher . . . E/G/S/T
39. Meditation and Gayatri . . . . S

175

40.	Mithila – A New Age Syllabus	E/G/S
41.	Nutana Yoga (New Age Yoga)	T
42.	Occult Meditations	E/G
43.	OM	T
44.	On Change *	E/G/S
45.	On Healing	E/G/S
46.	On Love *	E/G/S
47.	On Silence *	E/G/S
48.	Our Teacher and His Works	G/E
49.	Pranayama *	T
50.	Prayers	E
51.	Puranapurushuni Pooja Vidhanam	T
52.	Rudra	E/G/S
53.	Sai Suktulu	T
54.	Sankhya – The Sacred Doctrine	E/G/S
55.	Sankya Yoga	T
56.	Sarannavaratra Pooja Vidhanamu	T
57.	Saraswathi – The Word	E/G
58.	Saturn – The Path to Systematised Growth	E/G/S
59.	Shodosopachara Pooja - Avagahana	T
60.	Sound – The Key and its Application	E/S
61.	Spiritual Fusion of East and West *	E
62.	Spiritualism, Business and Management *	E/G/S
63.	Spirituality in Daily Life	S
64.	Sri Dattatreya	E/G/S/T/HI
65.	Sri Hanuman Chalisa	T

66.	Sri Krishna Namamrutham.	T
67.	Sri Lalitha I	T
68.	Sri Lalitha II	T
69.	Sri Mahalakshmi Pooja Vidhanamu	T
70.	Sri Sastry Garu	E/G/S/F/T
71.	Sri Shirdi Sai Sayings	E/G/S/T/HI
72.	Sri Siva Hridayamu	T
73.	Sri Soukumarya Satakam	T
74.	Sri Surya Pooja Vidhanamu	T
75.	Sri Venkateswara Pooja Vidhanamu	T
76.	Teachings of Lord Maitreya	T
77.	Teachings of Master Morya.	T
78.	Teachings of Master Devapi	T
79.	The Aquarian Cross	E/G/S
80.	The Aquarian Master	E/G/S
81.	The Doctrine of Ethics	E
82.	The Etheric Body *	E/G/S
83.	The Masters of Wisdom.	S
84.	The Path of Synthesis *	E
85.	The Splendor of Seven Hills *	E/T/HI
86.	The White Lotus *	E/G/S
87.	Theosophical Movement	E/G/S
88.	Time – The Key *	E/G/S
89.	Venus – The Path to Immortality	E/G/S
90.	Vinayaka Vratakalpamu.	T
91.	Vratakalpamu .	T

92. Vishnu Sahasranamam . . . . T
93. Vrutrasura Rahasyam . . . . T
94. Wisdom Buds * . . . . E/S
95. Wisdom Teachings of Vidura . . . . . E/G/S